FEEL BETTER, LIVE LONGER WITH VITAMIN B-3

D1738022

FEEL BETTER, LIVE LONGER WITH VITAMIN B-3

Nutrient Deficiency and Dependency

DR ABRAM HOFFER, MD, FRCP (C)
& DR HAROLD D. FOSTER, PhD

CCNM
PRESS

The authors thank Jo Mawdsley for her skillful and accurate typing of this book, making our task much more pleasant. The authors dedicate the book to Stanislav Petrov who, by thinking outside the box, saved the planet on September 26, 1983. On that day, Lt. Colonel Stanislav Petrov was in charge of the USSR's ballistic missile early warning system command centre. A malfunction, triggered by a strange cloud formation, indicated that the USA had launched a nuclear attack. According to the warning system, USA missiles would reach Soviet soil in 15 minutes. The alarm sounded and a red button flashing indicated to Petrov that it was his duty to launch the Soviet arsenal of nuclear missiles. Retaliation from the USA, Britain and France would have been virtually instantaneous and World War III would have been over almost as fast as it began. Pressing the red button would have killed every man, woman, and child on the planet. But Petrov refused to press the button without proof of detonation of the first US missile. As a result of his unreliability, his military career was finished and he now lives on small pension in Friazino, just outside Moscow.

The publisher does not advocate the use of any particular treatment program, but believes that the information presented in this book should be available to the public. The nutritional, medical, and health information in this book is based on the research, training, and personal experiences of the authors, and is true and complete to the best of their knowledge. However, this book is intended only as an informative guide for those wishing to know more about good health. It is not intended to replace or countermand the advice given by the reader's physician. The publisher and the authors are not responsible for any adverse effects of consequences from any of the suggestions made in this book. Because each person and each situation is unique, the publisher and the authors urge the reader to consult with a qualified professional before using any procedure where there is any question as to its appropriateness.

ISBN (10 digit) 1-897025-24-6 (13 digit) 978-1-897025-24-6

Edited by Bob Hilderley. Design by Sari Naworynski.
Printed and bound in Canada.

Published by CCNM Press Inc., 1255 Sheppard Avenue East, Toronto, Ontario M2K 1E2 Canada. www.ccnmpress.com

CONTENTS

INTRODUCTION

The world is now suffering from a global vitamin B-3 deficiency and dependency pandemic, which is perhaps more devastating than the scurvy pandemic that preceded the discovery of the benefits of eating foods containing vitamin C (ascorbic acid). Dr Linus Pauling, in his fundamental study of "orthomolecular" nutrition and in his celebrated book *Vitamin C and the Common Cold,* showed how the human body lost its ability during evolution to make certain nutrients, including vitamin C. Other primates, the guinea pig, and an Indian fruit-eating bat also lost their ability to make this vitamin.

Similarly, man is going through the process right now of losing the ability to make vitamin B-3 from tryptophan, as Dr Pauling and Dr Hoffer have suggested in their book *Healing Cancer* and as is documented in this book. Schizophrenics are a group of people who have gone far in this direction. As diets have become high-tech and the amount of vitamin B-3 has been lowered, individuals who no longer have the ability to convert enough tryptophan to vitamin B-3 are becoming sick. If we were to add 100 mg of niacinamide to every person's diet, there would be a major decrease in the incidence of schizophrenia and many other diseases, including cardiovascular and coronary disease, Huntington's and Parkinson's disease, Alzheimer's disease and senility, arthritis and certain addictions, stress disorders and various cancers, as well as the classic vitamin B-3 deficiency disease, pellagra.

There are two main forms of vitamin B-3, nicotinic acid, known medically as niacin, and nicotinamide, known medically as niacinamide. The term vitamin B-3 refers to these two substances and to the nicotinamide adenine dinucleotide system, NAD and NADH. NADH is the reduced form and is more active than NAD. The term vitamin B-3 deficiency means a deficiency of niacin, niacinamide, nicotinamide adenine dinucleotide (NAD), or its reduced derivative, NADH.

This book's authors are not suggesting that vitamin B-3 is the most important vitamin. By definition, all vitamins are essential to health. The most important one for any particular person is the one most lacking. The best test to determine this is clinical. If a person takes a vitamin and after a short time becomes healthier and feels better, then obviously that vitamin was needed. If there is no improvement, this may be because they are not short of that vitamin, because the dose taken was too small, or because there are additional nutrient deficiencies that have not yet been corrected.

Dr Roger Williams once compared the action of nutrients to a concert given by a symphony orchestra. The musicians play from the same score, following a conductor. The quality of the music depends upon each musician performing according to the way the music is written. Each instrument played according to the score is essential for a harmonious production. Vitamin B-3 is one of the essential components of nature's grand symphony, as performed by each cell of our bodies. By discussing only vitamin B-3, we are not down-playing or minimizing the significance of other nutrients. They are all essential, and for optimum cell function, they are needed in specific concentrations.

The history of medical invention and progress is one of anecdotes, as told to physicians by their patients, or as told by one doctor to another based upon their own experiences. Traditionally, case histories written by doctors, published in medical journals, provided the incentive for other physicians to test new ideas. Eventually, when a consensus developed, a new treatment became incorporated into the practice of medicine. During the past 50 years, however, the medical profession, in its attempt to become more scientific, began to doubt and, eventually, to dismiss anecdotes as valueless. Today, they are not considered scientific. Judgment based upon testing the validity of anecdotes has been replaced by a reliance on statistics. As a consequence, P<0.05 – the probability that the difference observed during double blind controlled experiments has less than a 5% probability of being due to chance – has become the most revered symbol in modern medicine, perhaps equivalent to $E = mc^2$, the Einstein equation. It is ironic that the point at which something becomes acceptably statistically significant, P<0.05, was selected arbitrarily by the founder of modern bio-statistical analysis. Sir R.A. Fisher (1890-1962), in his 1925 book *Statistical Method for Research Workers*, arbitrarily selected P=0.05 as the important statistical variable.

As a consequence, the public now pays more attention to anecdotes than the medical profession, which ignores or attacks the use of such patient histories. Several years ago Dr Hoffer was given a booklet published in the 18th century and written by a mother for her daughter when she married. This contained valuable recipes, including one for scurvy. The mother advised her daughter to use "scurvie grass" if she was suffering from the common symptoms of this disease. It was another decade before Dr James Lind, using a very simple, elegant experiment, proved that oranges and lemons also cured scurvy.

Case studies or anecdotes are superb teaching tools when described by eminent authors. This was illustrated by Professor Guerin-Tosh in his biography, *Living Proof: A Medical Mutiny*. He was stricken by myeloma, a deadly form of cancer. In this biography, he describes how he dealt with this diagnosis, eventually using only alternative methods, including nutrients and the Gerson therapy. He is alive and well 8 years later, despite the fact that the foremost experts in England told him he would be dead in 1 year if he did not take standard cancer treatment. This type of medical anecdote surely should be taken very seriously.

Of the diseases and disorders that appear related to vitamin B-3 deficiency and dependency, only the schizophrenia and cholesterol relationships have been assessed using double blind studies. The rest are based on careful observations by orthomolecular physicians. A single successfully tested case does not establish a treatment, but it does suggest that there may be others who would benefit from the same protocol. In every new treatment, there has to be the first case. If a patient is treated and recovers, there are several possibilities. First, the patient may be the only case any-where that could have reacted in this way. Second, the recovery had noth-ing to do with the treatment because it was entirely a placebo reaction. Third, the treatment works.

The first possibility is extremely rare. It is highly unlikely that only one person in the entire world with that condition would have responded to that treatment. It is much more probable that there are other patients who would benefit from the protocol. The second possibility is more likely. The solution to this dilemma is to try the same treatment on other patients. If a large percentage respond favorably, a placebo reaction can be ruled out. When case histories of recovered patients treated with vitamin B-3 are given in this book, it means that there are probably many others with the ailment who will also recover in the same way, but, as the research had not been done, it is as yet unclear what proportion of that population with the same disease will also be responsive.

It is our hope that the information provided here will generate enough interest in vitamin B-3 to ensure that the necessary additional studies will be completed. For each disease or condition examined, we provide the basic references to the literature which discusses the use of vitamin B-3 as a treatment, a brief summary of the results to be expected, and case histo-ries that illustrate what might be achieved.

Nutrient Deficiency and Dependency

SCAVENGING AND SYNTHESIZING

To survive, every species (including our own) requires a wide variety of essential nutrients. There are two distinct ways to obtain these substances. They can be internally synthesized in biochemical reactions or they can be scavenged externally from the environment – from water, soils, plants, or other species. Synthesis requires redirecting energy away from other bodily functions to the synthesizing activity. Scavenging is the driving force behind the evolution of longer necks, bigger jaws, stronger teeth, greater speed, more aggressive behavior, and other characteristics that may assist any species in the competition for scarce resources.

When a nutrient is hard to find or the supply is unreliable, there is a strong impetus within the species to synthesize it. Synthesis of nutrients appears to be a safest route to survival for a species. Relying on the milieu to provide a nutrient is a risky business in an environment with the potential for rapid change. The availability of a particular nutrient may vary significantly, which is one reason why the number of prey and predators rise and fall in unison.

Nevertheless, when a nutrient is readily available from the local environment, there is a tendency in the species to rely on direct scavenging.

Indeed, a species may gradually lose the ability to synthesize a nutrient when it is abundant in the environment.

However, obtaining nutrients for survival is not always an either/or proposition – either to scavenge or to synthesize. Species are typically in a state of flux. The situation may arise when the species can synthesize the nutrient to meet part of its need, but still scavenges the environment for the balance. The situation may also arise where the species can no longer synthesize the nutrient, and the nutrient is no longer abundant in the environment. This appears to have happened to humans in the case of vitamin C and is occurring today in the case of vitamin B-3.

Vitamin C Deficiency

Approximately 4,000 mammals can still synthesize vitamin C (ascorbic acid), producing, on average, some 50 mg of vitamin C per kg of body weight each day. Although humans have significant requirements for vitamin C, they cannot synthesize it and are forced to scavenge it from their environments. This dependency often leads to a deficiency, however, because humans typically ingest only 1 mg per kg of body weight of this vitamin daily.[1] That is, without supplementation, the environment no longer provides humans with the optimum intake of vitamin C. This dual inability to synthesize ascorbic acid or to acquire it in adequate quantity from the environment is associated with numerous deficiency diseases, the most famous being scurvy.

In 1741, the chaplain of the British warship *Centurion* described a serious outbreak of scurvy, providing insights into a wide spectrum of symptoms. The vessel was on its way around Cape Horn to the "South Sea," on a mission to attack Spanish colonies on the west coast of South America, during the War of Jenkin's Ear.[2]

...its [scurvy's] symptoms are inconstant and innumerable, and its progress and effects extremely irregular; for scarcely any two persons have the same complaints, and where there hath been found some conformity in the symptoms, the order of their appearance has been totally different. However, though its frequently puts on the form of many other diseases, and is therefore not to be described by any

exclusive and infallible criterions; yet there are some symptoms which are more general than the rest, and therefore, occurring the oftenest, deserve a more particular enumeration. These common appearances are large discoloured spots dispersed over the whole surface of the body, swelled legs, putrid gums, and above all, an extraordinary lassitude of the whole body, especially after any exercise, however inconsiderable; and this lassitude at last degenerates into a proneness to swoon on the least exertion of strength, or even on the least motion.

This disease is likewise usually attended with a strange dejection of the spirits, and with shiverings, tremblings, and a disposition to be seized with the most dreadful terrors on the slightest accident.

But it is not easy to complete the long roll of the various concomitants of this disease; for it often produced putrid fevers, pleurisies, the jaundice, and violent rheumatick pains, and sometimes it occasioned an obstinate costiveness, which was generally attended with a difficulty of breathing; and this was esteemed the most deadly of all the scorbutick symptoms: At other times the whole body but more especially the legs were subject to ulcers of the worst kind, attended with rotten bones, and such a luxuriancy of funguous flesh, as yielded to no remedy. But a most extraordinary circumstance, and what would be scarcely credible upon any single evidence is that the scars of wounds which had been for many years healed, were forced open again by this virulent distemper.

For hundreds of years, countless sailors died of scurvy on long sailing voyages.[3] Shipboard diet was boring, consisting of hardtack, salted meats, dried peas, fish, butter, cheese, beer, and fresh water. Generally, mariners ate enough food to meet their daily caloric needs, but lacking fruits and vegetables, their diet did not provide adequate ascorbic acid. The key issue was not food quantity but quality. This problem was compounded by copper cooking pots; this metal is antagonistic with vitamin C. Several years later in 1747, onboard the *HMS Salisbury*, John Lind discovered the value of oranges and lemons (which contain high levels of vitamin C) in managing scurvy. A booklet, written a decade earlier by a mother to be given to her daughter on her wedding day, included advice on what to do for "scurvie." The mother advised her daughter to use "scurvie" grass. Scurvie grass (spoonwort) has antiscorbutic properties.

Small amounts of vitamin C in our food can prevent scurvy. This does not mean that the inability of our species to synthesize ascorbic acid no longer has medical implications. The current Recommended Dietary Allowance (RDA) for vitamin C is 76 mg daily for males, 90 mg each day for females, and an additional 35 mg for smokers. This is the amount required to prevent scurvy and provide body stores for a month, with a margin of safety. It has been argued that "at 200 mg oral intake, blood plasma has more than 80% maximal concentration of vitamin C and tissues were completely saturated. Doses of 500 mg and higher are completely excreted in the urine."[4] For this reason, the National Institutes of Health investigators have maintained that five daily servings of vegetables and fresh fruits are enough to provide about 200 mg of ascorbic acid and so allow blood levels of vitamin C to reach their optimums. However, recent studies have shown this belief to be in error.[5]

As described in an *Annals of Internal Medicine* study, "When 3,000 milligrams [of ascorbic acid] was given orally every four hours, concentrations were nearly three times greater (220 micromole) than what was believed to be the maximum that could be achieved through oral consumption (70-85 micromole): single one gram supplement doses can produce transient plasma concentrations that are 2- to 3-fold higher than those from vitamin C-rich foods (200-300 mg daily)." In short, it is quite easy to cause plasma and tissue levels of ascorbic acid that are greater than what can be produced by eating vitamin C-enriched foods. To do this, supplements are required. Ingesting these mimic the high concentrations of vitamin C synthesized by almost all other mammals.

Apparently, it is easy to raise plasma and tissue levels of vitamin C, but is it necessary? Is the RDA for ascorbic acid incompetently low? The answer to both questions is obviously yes.

Throughout hundreds of thousands of years of evolution, humans became genetically adapted to their diets, lifestyles, and environments. However, since the advent of the Agricultural Revolution 9000 years ago and the Industrial Revolution a few centuries ago, the human diet has changed radically, but during this relatively short time period, virtually no new genetic adaptations have occurred. Indeed, humans today seem to be genetically identical to their pre-agricultural, Paleolithic ancestors, with the same demand for vitamins and minerals, but eat a different diet of predominantly processed foods. Pre-agricultural man ate a diet that contained vitamins and mineral levels that were several times higher than current RDA recommendations. The Paleolithic RDA ratio for vitamin C, for example, was approximately 6.7 higher. That is, the average Paleolithic diet probably provided almost seven times the current recommended daily allowance for ascorbic acid.

What then are the implications of underestimating human requirements for this vitamin? An epidemiological study, published in 2000 by the National Institutes of Health, showed that adults with blood plasma concentrations of more than 73.8 micromoles of vitamin C experienced a 57% reduction in risk of dying of any cause and 62% reduced relative risk of dying of cancer when compared with individuals consuming low amounts of vitamin C and having blood plasma concentrations of 28 micromoles or less.[6] A further study showed that, for every 500 microgram increase in blood serum vitamin C concentration, there was an 11% reduction in coronary heart disease and stroke prevalence.[7] Other diseases that seem to be occurring more frequently because of the human inability to synthesize vitamin C or get adequate amounts of it from diet (without supplementation) include arthritis, gall bladder disease, aortic aneurysm, and angina.

Vitamin B-3 Deficiency

The same principles hold true for vitamin B-3 (niacin). That is, pre-agricultural humans formerly ate a diet that provided them with an adequate intake of niacin. To save energy for other purposes, their ability to synthesize niacin from the amino acid tryptophan was very largely, but not entirely, lost. However, diets changed and foods are now often processed, such that the environment is no longer providing adequate niacin to the great majority of humanity. Unfortunately, synthesis cannot now make up for this deficiency, and a wide variety of illnesses result from this inadequacy. Fortunately, these diseases can be prevented and treated by niacin supplementation, just as scurvy, many cancers, heart disease, and stroke can be avoided by elevating vitamin C intake.

Pellagra, for example, at one time devastated the population of several countries and the Southern United States, where the population was dependent on corn as its staple food. Pellagra is characterized by four "Ds": diarrhea, dermatitis, dementia, and death, if not treated. Corn alone cannot meet our minimum need for vitamin B-3. For centuries, Central Americans have recognized from experience that treating maize with a lime solution before it is cooked reduced the onset of pellagra symptoms. Such an alkali solution releases niacin from its tightly bound source. In response to this deficiency and the potential for pellagra, very small amounts of vitamin B-3 (nicotinamide) have been added to flour since 1942, a supplementing practice that has almost eradicated classical pellagra.

Dogs and Cats

The vitamin B-3 requirements of many mammals, including the dog, can be met partly by the synthesis of this vitamin from tryptophan. However, the cat's ability to convert tryptophan to niacin is now negligible.[8] While cats normally do not need to be given vitamin C because they are able to synthesize adequate amounts, they require diets containing about 40 mg of niacin per kg of body weight each day.[9] This is very similar to the amount of vitamin C synthesized daily by most mammals, but not, of course, humans. Cats have more or less lost the ability to synthesize niacin and most get pre-formed niacin supplements in their diets. Cats eating niacin-deficient diets develop "black tongue" hemorrhagic diarrhea, anemia, and reddening and ulceration of the mucous membranes of the tongue and mouth. If this inadequacy is not corrected, emaciation and death eventually occur. Humans face similar diseases if their diets are vitamin B-3 deficient.

Vitamins-as-Prevention

How did the modern diet become so deficient in certain nutrients that we can no longer scavenge adequate amounts? Food processing would seem to be the chief cause, although depletion of soil nutrients may also be implicated. The more a food is processed, the less nutritious and even dangerous it is likely to be. Many essential nutrients are removed during processing, potentially causing nutrient deficiency diseases, while excess salt, sugar, colorings, and other unhealthy additives are used to replace them.

What can be done to compensate for these losses? Ironically, food processing science led to the discovery of the very vitamins needed to supplement our nutrient-poor diets. For example, the processing of white rice led to the discovery of vitamin B-1 (thiamine). Polishing brown rice removes the bran and germ, as well as most of the vitamin B-1 (thiamine). This thiamine deficiency can cause beriberi, a major problem for the Japanese Navy in the late nineteenth century. Sailors with beriberi were cured when they were given rice bran or whole rice. Even as late as 1940, the major source of B vitamins was rice bran extract. Soon after, manufacturers of white bread began supplementing their product with the thiamine (vitamin B-1), riboflavin (vitamin B-2), and niacin (vitamin B-3) stripped from the whole grain in the 'whitening' process.

Vitamin B-1 was the first B complex vitamin to be identified, followed by two other water soluble vitamins, vitamin B-2 and vitamin B-3. The B complex vitamins are very powerful, so only low quantities are needed to prevent deficiency diseases. For example, only 12 mg daily of vitamin B-3 is required to avoid developing pellagra.

Vitamins were now recognized as essential for preventing classic deficiency diseases, such as scurvy, beriberi, pellagra, rickets, some forms of pernicious anemia, and so on. Studies of deficiency diseases were very useful in helping scientists isolate these elusive substances. By 1950, the current range of the vitamins had been discovered and their structures determined. They also had been synthesized and were commercially available.

This vitamins-as-prevention paradigm was based upon the belief that vitamins were needed only in very small doses to prevent deficiency diseases. This is a partial truth. For the classical deficiency diseases, in every case, small amounts of the respective vitamin added to the diet in food or supplement form could prevent the disease from occurring. It followed that if vitamins are needed only in very small doses to prevent deficiency diseases, large doses are unnecessary. This belief that only small doses are required has been enshrined in the establishment of recommended daily allowances (RDAs) for most nutrients, adopted as nutrition guides by public health agencies in most Western nations.

Vitamins-as-Therapy

Soon after vitamins were established as preventive for many classic deficiency diseases, their role as therapeutic agents was discovered in treating disease using large doses. This was first recognized in the treatment of pellagra and schizophrenia.

In the early 1900s, one quarter of all spring-time admissions to mental hospitals in the southeastern United States were psychotic pellagrins who could not be distinguished from schizophrenics until they were given synthetic niacin. If they responded quickly to this vitamin, they were called pellagrins, and if they did not, they were termed schizophrenics. In the 1930s, researchers began to recognize that only patients who had recently developed pellagra recovered when given small, 10-mg, 'vitamin-sized' doses of vitamin B-3. If patients had been sick for a long time, they needed large doses of this vitamin, as high as 600 mg daily. However, the use of doses 60 times greater to treat chronic pellagra was inconsistent with the vitamin-as-prevention paradigm.

A decade later, Dr E. Shute and Dr W. Shute found that vitamin E, in large doses, was therapeutic for heart disease and for many cases of burns.[10, 11] They based their conclusions on thousands of patients they had treated, but unfortunately their work was derided at the time. Vitamin E had not yet been accepted as a vitamin, and it was "known" with certainty that vascular disease was not a vitamin deficiency disease. In 1960, researchers from Harvard University examined the Shutes' original data and protocols, reiterating the claim that vitamin E could not reverse vascular disease. Recent research has proven otherwise.

Also in the 1940s, Dr William Kaufman began to treat arthritis patients with large doses of niacinamide, publishing two books and several excellent papers on his successes.[12] Then, in the early 1950s, Dr Fred Klenner began to give his patients enormous doses of vitamin C, both orally and intravenously.[13, 14] He claimed that this treatment was able to help patients with very serious diseases, such as hepatic cancer and multiple sclerosis.

In 1955, Dr Hoffer and his colleagues published a brief report showing that controlled large doses of niacin lowered cholesterol levels.[15] Significantly, high cholesterol is not a vitamin deficiency disease, although niacin in very large doses can reduce it, compared to the amount needed to reverse pellagra in new patients. The association between cholesterol and niacin levels was soon corroborated at the Mayo Clinic by Dr William Parsons Jr.[16] This paper is now considered the first major revision of the vitamins-as-prevention paradigm to include vitamins-as-treatment.

Hoffer's research in niacin therapy for high cholesterol levels derived from his earlier work in treating schizophrenia. In 1952, he was the Director of Psychiatric Research in the Department of Public Health for the Province of Saskatchewan. This department was responsible for two large mental hospitals and a school for the mentally challenged, which together housed over 5,000 patients. One half were schizophrenics. At the time, there was no viable treatment for this illness; these patients could expect to spend the rest of their lives in such facilities. There was nothing unusual about this situation: 25% of admissions to Canadian hospitals were schizophrenics, almost all of whom were eventually committed to similar inadequate mental hospitals.

As documented in his book *Vitamin B-3 and Schizophrenia: Discovery, Recovery, Controversy,* Hoffer's interest in the use of niacin as a means of treating schizophrenic patients can be traced back to 1951 when Dr Humphry Osmond took up the position of medical director of the hospital at Weyburn, Saskatchewan, located about 70 miles south-east of the province's capital, Regina.[17] Earlier, Osmond had completed a study with Dr John Smythies, which compared the experiences associated with taking mescaline, an hallucinogen derived from natural sources, such as from the Mexican cactus peyote (*Lophophra spp.*), with symptoms of schizophrenia. While not identical, numerous similarities were identified between the two conditions. Osmond and Smythies hypothesized that schizophrenia might be caused by a similar hallucinogen. Mescaline resembles adrenaline in structure. Since schizophrenia was clearly associated with stress, it was postulated that such an hallucinogen might be linked, in some way, to adrenaline.

Discussion centered around this issue at the first meeting of the Saskatchewan Committee on Schizophrenia Research. Professor Vernon Woodford suggested that since adrenochrome, an oxidation product of adrenaline, was a known mitotic poison, perhaps it was the hallucinogen involved in schizophrenia. If so, some safe and inexpensive method of blocking its impact was required.

Hoffer had previously obtained a doctoral degree in biochemistry by studying the distribution of vitamin B-2 in wheat seedlings and, therefore, was familiar with the current literature on vitamins. The ability of niacin and niacinamide to prevent another serious mental illness, pellagra, appeared to be of great significance. Hoffer knew that niacin and niacinamide, collectively known as vitamin B-3, prevented pellagra and could also cure it in high doses.

There was little doubt that high doses of vitamin B-3 could be tolerated for long periods. Indeed, it had been shown that the LD_{50} in animals (the amount of the vitamin which, if given all at once, would cause the death of 50% of a group of test animals) was 4 g per kg. If humans reacted to vitamin B-3 in the same way as rats and other animals, then it would take roughly a 200 g dose to kill a 50 kg woman and 320 g to cause the death of an 80-kg man. Even these assumptions eventually were found to be untrue, since it is apparently almost impossible to take a fatal overdose of vitamin B-3.

Given the value of this vitamin in the treatment of pellagra and its very low toxicity, it was decided to begin some therapeutic trials using niacin and other nutrients to treat schizophrenia. Since the formation of adrenochrome involves an oxidation reaction, Hoffer and Osmond also decided to use high levels of an anti-oxidant to prevent its production. Ascorbic acid was the only anti-oxidant available at the time.

The first patient treated responded very positively. Ken, aged 21, was a chronic, violent, catatonic schizophrenic being treated at the hospital in Weyburn, where Osmond was medical director. He was admitted in February 1952 and given electroconvulsive therapy, which made him slightly better for a brief period. He then relapsed. He was given insulin to produce a coma, but gradually got worse. When Hoffer was delivering the first supply of pure niacin and ascorbic acid to Osmond, the chief psychiatrist told them that Ken was dying. The patient was in a catatonic coma. They decided to give him these two vitamins. There was nothing to lose and everything to gain, possibly a life.

They rushed to the ward and found Ken flat on his back breathing stertorously, unable to respond. He could not drink. They gave him, by a stomach tube, 5 g of niacin and 5 g of ascorbic acid dissolved in water, despite being unaware of any report describing the use of such a high dose of niacin. The next day Ken sat up and drank the dissolved vitamins himself. Fourteen days later he was normal. His family took him home 1 month after he had been given his first dose. About 13 years later, Hoffer traced this former patient and found him to be in good health, working as a contractor and serving as Chair of the Board of Trade in his town.

Orthomolecular Medicine

Since Hoffer's pioneering work with large doses of niacin for treating high cholesterol and schizophrenia, others have taken up the torch, showing the efficacy of niacin and other vitamins in treating a wide variety of diseases and disorders, none more notably than Dr Linus Pauling in his highly influential books *Vitamin C and the Common Cold* and *Cancer and Vitamin C* (co-authored with Dr Ewan Cameron).

Pauling coined the term 'orthomolecular' to describe the use of nutrients in large doses (megadoses) to treat specific conditions, including psychiatric conditions. In his ground-breaking article on "Orthomolecular Psychiatry," first published in *Science* magazine in 1968, Pauling stated that "orthomolecular therapy, consisting of the provision for the individual person of the optimum concentration of important normal constituents of the brain, may be the preferred treatment for many mentally ill patients."[18] He defined orthomolecular psychiatry as "the achievement and preservation of mental health by varying concentrations in the human body of substances that are normally present, such as vitamins. It is part of a broader subject, orthomolecular medicine, an important part because the functioning of the brain is probably more sensitively dependent in its molecular composition and structure than is the functioning of other organs." In *Healing Cancer*, co-authored with Dr Hoffer, Pauling added, "orthomolecular medicine is the prevention and treatment of disease by regulating the concentrations in the human body of orthomolecular substances."[19]

Dr Bernard Rimland, author of *Infantile Autism*, further explains the meaning of orthomolecular substances and contrasts the practice of 'orthomolecular' medicine with 'toximolecular' medicine: "'Ortho' means straight, or correct, and 'molecular' refers to the chemistry of the body. 'Orthomolecular' thus means correcting the chemistry of the body. To contrast the philosophies of establishment medicine and orthomolecular medicine, I have coined the word 'toximolecular' to refer to the common practice of trying to treat disease (or at least the symptoms of disease) through the use of toxic chemicals. It doesn't make much sense to me; it is dangerous, expensive, and not very effective. But it is profitable. Most vitamins are quite safe, in contrast to the drugs in widespread use, which can be and all too often are lethal in large amounts. Traditional medicine consists largely of giving lethal drugs in sub-lethal amounts, it seems to me. Orthomolecular psychiatry is not only much safer, it is much more sensible. Its emphasis on the use of substances normally present in the human really makes sense." [20]

Each cell in our body is a biochemical powerhouse in charge of thousands of reactions involving a myriad of compounds, all operating in harmony. The cell can grow, repair itself, and die on key. Plant cells are better at making important compounds. Give a plant cell minerals, sunlight, water, and a safe place to grow, and the lowly algae can make all the vitamins it needs. Animal cells are less versatile in meeting their requirements, but are more adept at using the fruits of the labors of the plant cells. Animals eat other animals and plants, but their major source of nutrients is plant life. If there is a deficiency of one of the important nutrients or compounds that the cell needs in order to function, the whole procedure slows or stops. Just as in a factory that assembles cars, if one vital part does not get delivered in time, the whole plant shuts down.

When a cell is not working properly because it is lacking an essential substance, that natural substance cannot be adequately replaced by a xenobiotic substance – that is, a chemical or drug that is foreign to the body. How will this allow the cell to regain its full function? Drugs are synthetics that are not naturally present in the body and for which the body does not have ready-made mechanisms for their destruction and elimination.

Imagine a modern orchestra with all the instruments working on the same beat and following the same music, under control of the conductor, when suddenly the first violinist is taken ill. Will the orchestra sound the same if the first violin is replaced by a drum? Xenobiotic compounds are not accepted by the body as natural substances. Orthomolecular substances are like instruments in their proper setting, while xenobiotics are like the drum inserted where it does not belong. The closer in structure a xenobiotic is to a natural substance, the more likely the body is to tolerate it, but the xenobiotic can never be used as fully as the natural substance it seeks to replace. That is why all the natural substances, including vitamins, minerals, hormones, amino acids, and essential fatty acids, are safer and more valuable in health care than are the xenobiotics drugs. This was the genius of Linus Pauling – he recognized this reality.

The practice of orthomolecular medicine thus recognizes that most acute and chronic diseases are due to a metabolic fault that is correctable in most patients by good nutrition, including the use of large doses of vitamins and mineral supplements. Unlike conventional medicine, orthomolecular medicine recognizes the principle of individuality, recommending the optimum diet of nutrients for each of us, in good health and in poor health. No two patients are the same; therefore, no two treatments are the same. Linus Pauling's orthomolecular approach proposes that people vary considerably, and their required intake of vitamins changes with their state of health. This is more biologically plausible than setting a fixed requirement for the entire population.

Orthomolecular medicine requires the application of both of these principles: biochemical individuality and the use of optimum doses (large doses if needed) of nutrients, including vitamins, minerals, and amino and essential fatty acids, in the maintenance of good health and treatment of health conditions .

Vitamin Dependency

In contrast to a vitamin deficiency, where the diet does not offer enough of a nutrient to satisfy the needs of the average person, a dependency arises when the diet contains enough of the nutrient for the average person, but not enough for certain patients with extremely high requirements.

The words deficiency and dependency lie at opposite ends of a continuum of need, which ranges from very small to very large, a continuum stretching from the vitamins-as-prevention paradigm to the vitamins-as-treatment paradigm.

As Andrew W. Saul explains this principle of vitamin dependency in an article published in the *Journal of Orthomolecular Medicine*, "dependency is a fact of life. The human body is dependent on food, water, sleep, and oxygen. Additionally, its internal chemistry is absolutely dependent on vitamins. Without adequate vitamin intake, the body will sicken; virtually any prolonged vitamin deficiency is fatal. Surely this constitutes a dependency in the generally accepted sense of the word. "Nutrient deficiency of long standing may create an exaggerated need for the missing nutrient, a need not met by dietary intakes or even by low-dose supplementation. Recently, Robert P. Heaney, M.D., used the term 'long latency deficiency diseases' to describe illnesses that fit this description.[21] He writes: 'Inadequate intakes of many nutrients are now recognized as contributing to several of the major chronic diseases that affect the populations of the industrialized nations. Often taking many years to manifest themselves, these disease outcomes should be thought of as long-latency deficiency diseases. . . Inadequate intakes of specific nutrients may produce more than one disease, may produce diseases by more than one mechanism, and may require several years for the consequent morbidity to be sufficiently evident to be clinically recognizable as 'disease.' Because the intakes required to prevent the respective index diseases, recommendations based solely on preventing the index diseases are no longer biologically defensible.'

"There are at least two key concepts presented here. The first is, 'Inadequate intakes of specific nutrients may produce more than one disease.' This exactly supports Dr William Kaufman's statements to this effect 55 years ago, when he wrote that, in considering 'different clinical entities one cannot exclude the possibility that they may be caused by the same etiologic agent, acting in different ways. For example, in experimental animals, it has been shown that the lack of a single essential nutrient can produce a variety of dissimilar clinical disorders in different individuals of the same species. One might not suspect that the same etiologic factor, lack of a specific essential nutrient, was responsible for each of the various clinical syndromes of the same tissue deficiency disease which is permitted to develop at different rates in different individuals of the same species.'

"While amyotrophic lateral sclerosis, progressive muscular atrophy, progressive bulbar palsy, and primary lateral sclerosis are not all the same illness, they and the other neuromuscular diseases may have a common basis: unacknowledged, untreated long-term vitamin dependency. Therefore, each may respond to an orthomolecular approach, such as that successfully used by Dr Frederick R. Klenner for multiple sclerosis and myasthenia gravis half a century ago.

"The second key point Dr Heany makes is that vitamin 'intakes required to prevent many of the long-latency disorders are higher than those required to prevent the respective index diseases.' This confirms Dr Abram Hoffer's observations to this effect some 40 years ago, when he treated prisoners of war presenting severe, protracted nutrient deficiencies. Dr Hoffer wrote that when released, after as much as 44 months of captivity, 'only 75% had survived.[22] They had lost about one-third of their body weight. In camp they suffered from classical scurvy, beriberi, pellagra, many infections, and from protein and calorie deficiency. They were rehabilitated in hospitals and were given doses of vitamins that were then considered high. Since then these Hong Kong veterans have suffered from a variety of physical and psychiatric conditions.' However, 'the history of a small sample, about 12, is much different, for they have been taking nicotinic acid (niacin) 3 grams per day. These 12 have recovered and remain well as long as they take this quantity of vitamin regularly.'

"About 35 years ago (in the 1930s and 1940s) it was reported that some chronic pellagrins required at least 600 mg per day of vitamin B-3 to prevent the return of pellagra symptoms. This was astonishing then and unexplainable since pellagra as a nicotinic acid deficiency disease should have yielded to vitamin (small) doses. Today the concept of vitamin-dependency disease has developed. It is based upon the realization that there is a much wider range of need for nutrients than was believed to be true then.

"A person is said to be vitamin dependent if his requirements for that vitamin are much greater (perhaps 100-fold greater or more) than is the average need for any population. The optimum need is that quantity which maintains the subject in good health, not that quantity which barely keeps him free of pellagra. From this point of view, the Hong Kong veterans have become vitamin B-3 dependent as a result of severe and prolonged malnutrition. It is likely that any population similarly deprived of essential nutrients for a long period of time will develop one or more dependency conditions.

"Thirty years ago, in another paper, Dr Hoffer stated that 'the newer concept of vitamin-dependent disease changes the emphasis from simply dietary manipulation to consideration of the endogenous needs of the organism.[23] It comes within the field of orthomolecular disease. The borderline between vitamin-deficiency and vitamin-dependency conditions is merely a quantitative one when one considers prevention and cure.'

"The differentiation between deficiency and dependency is dose. Every patient who was ever helped by high-dose nutrient therapy lends support to the concept of vitamin dependency. By the same token, symptoms result-ing from inappropriate and abrupt termination of large doses of nutrients provide equally good evidence for vitamin dependency. While deprivation of low doses of vitamin C causes scurvy, abrupt termination of high main-tenance doses may cause its own set of problems. Called 'rebound scurvy', this includes classical scorbutic symptoms, as well as a predictable relapse of illness that had already responded to high-dose therapy.

"As Robert F. Cathcart, M.D., notes, 'there is a certain dependency on ascorbic acid that a patient acquires over a long period of time when he takes large maintenance doses. Apparently, certain metabolic reactions are facili-tated by large amounts of ascorbate and if the substance is suddenly with-drawn, certain problems result such as a cold, return of allergy, fatigue, etc. Mostly, these problems are a return of problems the patient had before taking the ascorbic acid. Patients have by this time become so adjusted to feeling better that they refuse to go without ascorbic acid. Patients do not seem to acquire this dependency in the short time they take doses to bowel tolerance to treat an acute disease. Maintenance doses of 4 grams per day do not seem to create a noticeable dependency. The majority of patients who take over 10-15 grams of ascorbic acid per day probably have certain meta-bolic needs for ascorbate, which exceed the universal human species need. Patients with chronic allergies often take large maintenance doses.'[24]

"The major problem feared by patients benefiting from these large maintenance doses of ascorbic acid is that they may be forced into a posi-tion where their body is deprived of ascorbate during a period of great stress such as emergency hospitalization. Physicians would recognize the consequences of suddenly withdrawing ascorbate under these circum-stances and be prepared to meet these increased metabolic needs for ascor-bate in even an unconscious patient. These consequences of ascorbate depletion which may include shock, heart attack, phlebitis, pneumonia, allergic reactions, increased susceptibility to infection, etc., may be averted only by ascorbate. Patients unable to take large oral doses should be given intravenous ascorbate. All hospitals should have supplies of large amounts of ascorbate for intravenous use to meet this need.

"This need is especially serious for the cancer patient, whose exceptionally positive response to mega-ascorbate therapy, and dramatically negative response to ascorbate deprivation, is the very picture of vitamin dependency.

"As Linus Pauling's colleague Ewan Cameron, M.D., wrote, 'ascorbate, however administered, is rapidly excreted in the urine, so that administration should be continuous or at very frequent intervals. Furthermore, exposure to high circulating levels of ascorbate induces over-activity of certain hepatic enzymes concerned with its degradation and metabolism. These enzymes persist for some time after sudden cessation of high intakes, resulting in depletion of circulating levels of ascorbate to well below normal unsupplemented values. This is known as the rebound effect. It causes a sharp decrease in immunocompetence and must be avoided in the cancer patient. Clinical experience has shown that the best responses are observed when vitamin C is administered intravenously, so insuring a high plasma level. However, because long-term continuous intravenous administration is impractical, we recommend an initial intravenous course of ten days duration, followed by continuous maintenance oral regimen.'[25]

"In short, the body only misses what it needs. That is dependency. The destructive consequences of alcohol and other negative drug dependencies are taught in elementary schools. At the same time, the consequences of ignoring our positive nutrient dependencies go largely undiscussed, even in medical journals. Vitamin dependencies induced by genetics, diet, drugs, or illness are most often regarded as medical curiosities. The Hoffer-Osmond discovery that schizophrenics, forming about 1% or 2% percent of the population, are dependent on multi-gram doses of niacin remains a psychiatric heresy. The Irwin Stone-Linus Pauling idea of population-wide, genetically-based hypoascorbemia has received negative attention, when it has received any attention at all. Yet, writes Dr Emanual Cheraskin, 'hypovitaminosis C is a very real and common, probably epidemic, problem, which clearly has not been properly viewed and surely not adequately reported.'[26] This is not a total surprise. It took decades for medical acknowledgment that biotin and vitamin E are actually essential to health.

"Simple cause-and-effect micronutrient deficiency, a doctrine long enamored of by the dietetic profession, is not always sufficient to explain persistent physician reports of megavitamin cures of a number of diseases outside the classically accepted few. Perhaps it is a law of orthomolecular therapy that the reason one nutrient can cure so many different illnesses is because a deficiency of one nutrient can cause many different illnesses.

"And if nutrient deficiency is basically about inadequate intake, then dependency is essentially about heightened need. As a dry sponge soaks up more milk, so a sick body generally takes up higher vitamin doses. The quantity of a nutritional supplement that cures an illness indicates the patient's degree of deficiency. It is, therefore, not a megadose of the vitamin, but rather a megadeficiency of the nutrient that we are dealing with. Orthomolecular practitioners know that with therapeutic nutrition, you don't take the amount that you believe ought to work; rather, you take the amount that gets results. The first rule of building a brick wall is that you have got to have enough bricks. A sick body has exaggeratedly high needs for many vitamins. We can either meet that need, or else suffer unnecessarily.

"Until the medical professions fully embrace orthomolecular treatment, 'medicine' might well be said to be 'the experimental study of what happens when poisonous chemicals are placed into malnourished human bodies.'"

Biochemical Individuality

The optimum intake of a nutrient varies enormously from patient to patient, depending on age, gender, disease, and other variables. For vitamin B-3, there is a continuum of need that ranges from the low doses that prevent pellagra to the very high doses that may be needed to reduce cholesterol levels. The same principle applies to other vitamins used as prevention and treatment.

Response to increasing doses is not linear; it is curvilinear. If the intake is very low, small doses will have a major impact. If the mean dose is higher, additional doses will have a less significant improvement effect. Once the optimum dose is reached, adding more will not improve the patient and may begin to cause side effects. Each disease will have its own dose response curve. That is why the Recommended Daily Allowances are of little therapeutic value. We need a specific RDA range for each condition and for each person because some people have a need for more than the deficiency level of a nutrient. They are dependent on a larger amount to be healthy.

Genetic Logic

Genes are the blueprints that allow for the production of proteins, which, in turn, are required to create, among other things, enzymes. However, slight variations in specific genes, known as alleles, occur from one individual to another. As a consequence, many genes carry two, several, or even many distinct variants of the same genetic information. Accordingly, even apparently very similar people may have distinct genetic information in specific genes. While some of these slight differences cause only minor variations in information and do not significantly affect health, others can have profound impacts.[27]

In a research study published in the *American Journal of Clinical Nutrition*, B.N. Ames and coworkers point out that as many as one-third of such genetic mutations seem to create enzymes that have decreased binding activities for their coenzymes.[28] This results in an enzyme that is less reactive than normal, making the carrier more susceptible to the disease or disorders associated with deficiencies of this specific enzyme.

Genes, however, are not necessarily destiny, as Ames explains: "About 50 human genetic diseases due to defective enzymes can be remedied or ameliorated by the administration of high doses of the vitamin component of the corresponding coenzyme, which at least partially restores enzymatic activity. Several single-nucleotide polymorphisms, in which the variant amino acid reduces coenzyme binding and thus enzymatic activity, are likely to be remediable by raising cellular concentrations of the cofactor through high-dose vitamin therapy."[29]

Simply put, there are many people who carry genetic mutations that require them to eat a diet abnormally high in a specific nutrient. If they do not, they will be unable to manufacture effective levels of a particular enzyme and, therefore, will be very likely to develop associated deficiency diseases. For such individuals, high specific vitamin or mineral supplements, well above the Recommended Daily Allowance, are not a luxury or a health threat – they are essential. In some cases, they require one thousand or more times the RDA amount.

Ames and coworkers have methodically provided details of a wide variety of such coenzyme decreased binding affinity diseases and the nutrients most likely to ameliorate them. For example, the enzyme cystathionine β-synthase catalyzes homocysteine and serine to form cystathionine. Individuals with a defective form of this enzyme develop very high blood and urine homocysteine levels that can cause a variety of symptoms, including mental retardation, vascular and skeletal problems, and optic lens dislocation. It has been found that roughly one half of cystathionine β-synthase deficient patients respond well to very high doses of vitamin B-6, the coenzyme for cystathionine β-synthase, which can lower their homocysteine and serine concentrations to normal levels.[30]

In most people, after a stiff drink or two of alcohol, the enzyme alcohol dehydrogenase oxidizes ethanol to acetaldehyde. The oxidation of this chemical is then catalyzed by a second enzyme, aldehyde dehydrogenase (NAD^+). However, some people have a naturally occurring variant of aldehyde dehydrogenase coded by the Lys487 allele. This particular version of the gene produces a form of aldehyde dehydrogenase that has only 8% of normal enzymatic function and an extremely reduced binding activity for its coenzyme, NAD. As a result, people with this allele cannot handle their alcohol consumption because they are genetically incapable of normal oxidation of acetaldehyde, which, therefore, builds up in their blood. This greatly increases their susceptibility to alcoholism, as well as to oral, esophageal, and stomach cancers, alcohol-induced vasospastic angina, and Alzheimer's disease.[31]

The key to dealing with this defective allele appears to be the administration of nicotinic acid or nicotinamide, both of which have been shown to increase intracellular NAD concentrations. Indeed, a 6-year Italian case-control study involving more than 1,000 participants has found that esophageal cancer risk was inversely correlated to niacin intake.[32] Not surprisingly, many alcoholics respond extremely well to high dose niacin treatment.

Other enzymes known to use NAD or niacin as a cofactor include glucose-6-phosphate 1-dehydrogenase, Complex 1, dihydropteridine reductase, and long-chain-3-hydroxyacyl-CoA dehydrogenase.[33] Alleles, genetic variants that produce aberrant enzymes with abnormally low efficacy, are known to be linked to greatly increased disease risk. Inefficient glucose-6-phosphate 1-dehydrogenase, for example, seems associated with hemolytic anemia and favism. Complex 1 abnormalities seem to be associated with elevated blood lactate and pyruvate. One allele of dihydropteridine reductase is known to be a key risk factor in phenylketonuria and cognitive dysfunction. A defective allele for long-chain-3-hydroxyacyl-CoA dehydrogenase seems linked to β-Oxidation defect, hypoglycemia, cardiomyopathy and sudden death.[34] Obviously, since all of these enzymes require NAD or niacin as a cofactor, the initial treatment protocol should involve high doses of vitamin B-3.

Revising RDAs

T he United States Food and Nutrition Board has prepared daily recommended nutrient allowances since 1941. Initially, they were based on the amount of vitamin C needed to prevent scurvy, which can easily be measured in short-term studies. The dose required to prevent acute scurvy was established many years ago as a few milligrams per day. However, the possibility remains that such low levels of vitamin C will not be enough to avoid longer-term deficiency diseases. Perhaps because this hypothesis is very difficult to test, it has largely been overlooked.

The Food and Nutrition Board ignores these possible long-term effects of nutrient inadequacy by claiming that there is no scientific proof that such diseases result from its recommendations. However, since science is based on refutation rather than proof, such a statement can always be made, no matter how strong the evidence. Just as an accused person is innocent until proven guilty, a scientific idea remains plausible until it has been shown to be incorrect. True scientists understand that "inadequate scientific proof" is often simply a fancy way of saying "we don't like this idea."

In the United States, the RDA is defined as the level of intake of essential nutrients that, on the basis of scientific knowledge, are judged by the Food and Nutrition Board to be adequate to meet the known nutrient needs of practically all healthy persons.[35] The RDA is said to be the amount of vitamin that provides the least risk of inadequacy and the least risk of toxicity. These adequacy and toxicity levels were not determined scientifically, however. Nevertheless, they persist because they provide a simple intake level that generally prevents acute deficiency.

Two important points are worth noting. First, most RDA standards are based on extrapolated data, which means they were not measured in actual experiments on real people. Second, even the experimental data collected from 19- to 30-year-old subjects was based on neutrophils, a white blood cell type that is known to have unusual vitamin C biochemistry, along with an exceptional ability to pump the vitamin into the cell body. The vitamin need of this cell type is not a reliable model for the body as a whole. The number of subjects used in the experiments on which the vitamin C recommendations were based was too small (15 males and 7 females) to allow an estimate of true biochemical variability in requirements. Indeed, the research involved only young, healthy subjects. Older, less healthy people might need more vitamin C – how much more was never examined.

Stressed and even mildly ill people can tolerate 10,000 times more vitamin C, implying a change in biochemistry that was ignored by those creating the RDA. The RDA concept also does not differentiate between short- and long-term effects of deprivation, yet the possibility that sub-clinical scurvy causes chronic disease has enormous implications for health. In summary, while setting the RDA for this vitamin, unsubstantiated risks of taking too much vitamin C have been accorded great importance, whereas the risks associated with not taking enough have been ignored.

In their book, *Ascorbate: The Science of Vitamin C,* Dr Hilary Roberts and Dr Steve Hickey concluded that RDAs for vitamin C are much too low.[36] "When the US and other governments decided on the recommended daily intake (RDA) for vitamin C, they used the best evidence available at the time. The question 'How much vitamin C does a healthy person need?' sounds relatively straightforward. In reality, the science behind this question is sophisticated and the evidence supporting the RDA has now been shown to be wrong. Consequently, the recommended intake of vitamin C could be less than a tenth of what we need. If people conform to the current recommendations, they may suffer long-term disease. Furthermore, there is no clear mechanism for the RDA to be modified when new scientific evidence emerges. Until revising the RDA is seen as more than an administrative inconvenience, people are likely to continue developing deficiency-based illnesses."

In sum, the arguments for the recommended daily allowances are barely justifiable as tentative suggestions, but they have been presented as having the authority of scientific laws. The RDA values were initially based on unscientific assumptions. The values are not justifiable in terms of genetics, biochemistry, or statistics. It is simply not sensible to recommend a single value for a varied population given the range of individual nutrient deficiency and dependency. Rather than recommended collective minimum daily allowances we need recommended individualized optimum allowances.

Determining Deficiency and Dependency

S till, no one knows how much of any given nutrient an individual human being requires to maintain good health or treat ill health. Despite a wide variety of opinions on optimum doses, the question remains open.

Ideally, we should have assay methods for determining whether patients are deficient in or dependent on a particular nutrient, but such technologies are not yet available. Reliable saturation tests will likely be developed eventually. Patients would be given various doses of a vitamin, with the amount excreted and the amount retained (and for how long) being measured. Current nutrient blood assays lack standard values for comparison. In contrast, for such substances as sugar or uric acid, large numbers of 'healthy' people are tested to obtain a normal distribution curve.

In the case of nutrient levels, the accuracy of this curve depends on the population being sampled. If half the sample is low in a certain nutrient and this population is used to prepare the standard values, then these values merely reinforce the erroneous idea that this population is not deficient in the nutrient. To prepare an accurate distribution curve, only people who are not deficient in that nutrient would need to be used. Today, that would be impossible. We do not recommend blood tests for vitamins, even for B-12 and folic acid, for that reason.

While there is no simple experiment or practical study that can rigorously provide an answer to how much of a given nutrient an individual needs to be healthy, some empirical guidelines can be followed. Orthomolecular physicians can rely upon their clinical judgment and patients' reports. Because these nutrients are safe, trial and error is an economical way of determining the optimum individual patient dose. For any given person, the amount of a nutrient needed is a result of a cost-benefit analysis. In the case of vitamin C, there appears to be little toxicity from high doses, which offer the promise of extended health and resistance to many chronic diseases. The costs of vitamin C supplementation are low, while the potential benefits are high. By contrast, the health costs of sticking to the low RDA could be enormous, whereas the benefits are minimal.

A new scientific theory, called the dynamic flow model, provides another guideline. According to this model, people should ideally be in a state of dynamic flow, which means they ingest more nutrient than they need so that any excess flows through the body and is excreted in the urine. The nutrient not normally required acts as a reservoir when extra quantities are required. For example, in the case of vitamin C, after a bee sting or at the start of a cold, more vitamin C is readily available to be absorbed from the gut.

The maximum burn-rate of vitamin C can be determined by increasing intake to bowel tolerance. To be in dynamic flow, one would need doses totalling half or more of the person's normal bowel tolerance level. The actual minimum daily requirement for optimum health could vary in the range of 100 mg to over 20 g (20,000 mg), depending on the individual. Because vitamin C is excreted quickly, the supplement should be divided into four or more daily doses. If the person developed an illness, the bowel tolerance level might also change quickly.

Dynamic flow is the closest humans can get to restoring their physiology to the way it was before they lost the ability to synthesize vitamin C. With modifications, the same model may be extended to determining the deficiency and dependency levels for other nutrients.

Multiple Nutrient Deficiency and Dependency

Dr David Horrobin, in the *British Journal of Nutrition*, has challenged the medical profession to apply these principles of nutrient deficiency and dependency in clinical practice. "Let's be imaginative and give multi nutrient supplementation a chance," he states. "We may already have most of the knowledge required to produce huge improvements in human health. To test the proposition, we may have to abandon two failed notions, the holistic one that we need to change diets, and the reductionist one that we should initially study single nutrients. If we do that, and if we incorporate the new findings on genetic variations in nutrient requirements, we could truly be at the beginning of one of the biggest and safest healthcare revolutions." [37]

References

[1] Ely J.T. Aneurysm: prevention and nonsurgical repair. Medical Science Monitor 2004;10(1): HY1 - HY4.

[2] Walter R. Extract from A Voyage Round the World in Rosenbaum, R.A. (ed). Best Book of True Sea Stories. New York, NY: Doubleday, 1966:143-51.

[3] Scurvy: Scourge of the Voyagers. Pathfinders and Passageways. The Exploration of Canada. Library and Archives Canada. http://www.collectionscanada.ca/exploreres/h24-1402-e.html

[4] National Institutes of Health News Release, April 20, 1999. NIH Research shows 100 to 200 mg of vitamin C daily may benefit healthy adults. http:www.nih.gov/news/pr/apr99/niddk-20.htm

[5] Gupta C. Share the Wealth Newsletter. The Vitamin C Fanatics Were Right All Along. July 09, 2004. http://www.newmediaexplorer.org/chris/2004/07/09/the_vitamin_c_fanatics_were_right.html

[6] Loria M, Klag MJ, Caulfield LE, Whelton PK. Vitamin C status and mortality in US adults. Am J Clin Nutr. 2000 July;72(1):139-45.

[7] Simon JA, Hudes ES, Browner WS. Serum ascorbic acid and cardiovascular disease prevalence in US adults. Epidemiology 1999 May;9(3):316-21.

[8] ADVANCE. Module 6.1 Special Requirements of Cats. http://www.speedyvet.com/nutrition/default.asp?module=6&page=specialrequirements

[9] Friis H. Micronutrients and infections: An introduction. In: Friis H (ed.) Micronutrients and HIV Infection. Boca Raton: CRC Press, 2001:1-21.

[10] Shute WB. Vitamin E Book. New Canaan, CT: Keats Publishing, 1978.

[11] Shute EV. The Heart and Vitamin E. London, ON: The Shute Foundation for Medical Research, 1969.

[12] Kaufman W: The common form of joint dysfunction: Its incidence and treatment. Brattleboro, VT: E.L. Hildreth and Co., 1949: http://www.doctoryourself.com;kaufman10.html.

[13] Klenner F. The treatment of poliomyelitis and other virus diseases with vitamin C. Journal of Southern Medicine and Surgery 1949;113:101-07.

[14] Smith L: Vitamin C as a fundamental medicine: Abstracts of Dr. Frederick R. Klenner, M.D.'s Published and Unpublished Work. Tacoma, WA: Life Sciences Press. 1988; renamed in 1991: Clinical Guide to the Use of Vitamin C: The Clinical Experiences of Frederick R. Klenner, M.D.

[15] Altschul R, Hoffer A, Stephen JD: Influence of nicotinic acid on serum cholesterol in man. Arch Biochem Biophys 1955;54:558-59.

[16] Parsons WB Jr. Cholesterol Control without Diet. The Niacin Solution. Revised, Expanded, 2nd ed. Scottsdale, AZ: Lilac Press, 2003.

[17] Hoffer A. Vitamin B-3 and Schizophrenia: Discovery, Recovery, Controversy. Kingston, ON: Quarry Health Books, 1998.

[18] Pauling L. Orthomolecular psychiatry. Science 1968;160:265-71.

[19] Hoffer A, Pauling L. Healing Cancer: Complementary Vitamin & Drug Treatments. Toronto, ON: CCNM Press, 2004.

[20] Rimland B. Recent research in infantile autism. Journal of Operational Psychology 1972;3:35;rpt.Autism Research Review International 1993;2.

[21] Heaney RP. Long-latency deficiency disease: Insights from calcium and vitamin D. Am J Clin Nutr. 2003 Nov;78(5):912-19.

[22] Hoffer A. Editorial. J. Orthomolecular Psychiatry 1974;3(1):34-36.

[23] Hoffer A. Mechanism of action of nicotinic acid and nicotinamide in the treatment of schizophrenia. In: Hawkins D and Pauling L (eds.). Orthomolecular Psychiatry: Treatment of Schizophrenia. San Francisco, CA: W.H. Freeman, 1973; 7:1359-76.

[24] Cathcart RF: Vitamin C, titration to bowel tolerance, anascorbemia, and acute induced scurvy. Medicine Hypothesis 1981;7:1359-76.

[25] Cameron E. Protocol for the use of vitamin C in the treatment of cancer. Medical Hypotheses 1991;36:190-94. Also: Cameron E: Protocol for the use of intravenous vitamin C in the treatment of cancer. Palo Alto, CA: Linus Pauling Institute of Science and Medicine,1986.

[26] Cheraskin E. Vitamin C and fatigue. J. Orthomolecular Medicine 1994;9:39-45

[27] Hartl DL, Freifelder D, Synder LA. Basic Genetics. Boston, MA: Jones and Bartlett, 1988:12.

[28] Ames BN, Elson-Schwab I, Silver EA. High-dose vitamin therapy stimulates variant enzymes with decreased coenzyme binding affinity (increased K_m): Relevance to genetic disease and polymorphisms. Am J Clin Nutr 2002;75:616-58.

[29] Ames BN, Elson-Schwab I, Silver EA. High-dose vitamin therapy stimulates variant enzymes with decreased coenzyme binding affinity (increased K_m): Relevance to genetic disease and polymorphisms. Am J Clin Nutr 2002;75:616-58.

[30] Barber GW, Spaeth GL. The successful treatment of homocystinuria with pyridoxine. J. Pediatr 1969;75:463-78.

[31] Ames BN, Elson-Schwab I, Silver EA. High-dose vitamin therapy stimulates variant enzymes with decreased coenzyme binding affinity (increased Km): Relevance to genetic disease and polymorphisms. Am J Clin Nutr 2002;75:632-37

[32] Franceschi S, Bidol E, Negri E, et al. Role of macronutrients, vitamins and minerals in the etiology of squamous-cell carcinoma of the oesophagus. Int. J. Cancer 2000;86:626-31.

[33] Ames BN, Elson-Schwab I, Silver EA. High-dose vitamin therapy stimulates variant enzymes with decreased coenzyme binding affinity (increased Km): Relevance to genetic disease and polymorphisms. Am J Clin Nutr 2002;75:632-37

[34] Ames BN, Elson-Schwab I, Silver EA. High-dose vitamin therapy stimulates variant enzymes with decreased coenzyme binding affinity (increased Km): Relevance to genetic disease and polymorphisms. Am J Clin Nutr 2002;75:632-37

[35] Nutrition Dictionary
http://www.foodfit.com/healthy/nutritionaldictionary.asp

[36] Roberts H, Hickey S. Ascorbate: The Science of Vitamin C.
www.lulu.com/ascorbate

[37] Horrobin D. Why do we not make more medical use of nutritional knowledge? How an inadvertent alliance between reductionist scientists, holistic dietitians and drug-oriented regulators and governments has blocked progress. British Journal of Nutrition 2003;90:233-38.

NIACIN DEFICIENCY PANDEMIC

A goat weighing as much as a typical man will normally synthesize about 14 g of vitamin C each day. Levels can rise if the animal is severely stressed. Indeed, most creatures can make all the vitamin C that they require. In contrast, humans cannot, despite the fact that this vitamin is absolutely essential for health. Linus Pauling discussed at length how this loss, by humans, of the ability to synthesize ascorbic acid probably conferred an initial evolutionary advantage that was so beneficial that it eventually spread throughout humanity, some apes, and a few other animals.[1,2] Certainly, the energy that this genetic aberration saved by not converting glucose into ascorbic acid could be used in other biochemical reactions, which probably increased mankind's ability to survive. Adverse consequences of this genetic change only became apparent when the food supply provided inadequate ascorbic acid.

This negative dietary change apparently occurred when humans descended from the trees onto the plains, migrating to regions of the planet where the vegetation contained lower levels of vitamin C. Irwin Stone, for example, has argued that all humans now naturally suffer from hypoascorbemia, a pandemic vitamin C deficiency disorder, also known as subclinical scurvy.[3] Stone considered that vitamin C was not simply a vitamin, but that it was an essential nutrient, with the same status as an amino acid.

A similar process has affected the synthesis of niacin, providing humans with both evolutionary advantages and disadvantages. Niacin is not a true vitamin in the strictest sense of the term because it can be produced in the body from the amino acid tryptophan. Nevertheless, the synthesis of niacin from tryptophan is a very inefficient process: 60 mg of the amino acid are necessary to provide 1 mg of niacin. This process also involves vitamins B-1, B-2, and B-6. If these are in short supply, the synthesis of vitamin B-3 will be even less efficient. Tryptophan itself is not usually readily available in diet, especially in those eating high levels of maize.[4]

While humans have the ability to synthesize niacin, this process is ineffective and is probably in evolutionary decline. Of course, vitamin B-3 is also available from many foods. If the diet contained enough of this vitamin to supply bodily requirements, then there would be no need to convert tryptophan to niacin. This would liberate energy for other uses, and free up tryptophan for the production of serotonin, a major neurotransmitter. Humanity would appear to be depending more and more on vitamin B-3 derived from diet, but recently niacin has become less available from food. As a result, subclinical pellagra and other niacin deficiency disorders are becoming very widespread.

Niacin Deficiency Prevalence

There is a great deal of evidence to support this argument. Approximately 50% of the population of the developed world seems to suffer from disorders or diseases that respond beneficially to niacin or niacinamide supplementation. This figure is probably an underestimate since those with arthritis (20%), addictions (10%), schizophrenia (2%), learning and/or behavioral disorders (5% of children), cardiovascular disease, coronary disease, and stroke (30%), cancer (50%), or severe stress (unknown) would very likely improve if given more niacin. The addition of 100 mg of niacinamide to the public diet would enormously reduce human suffering and have a major impact on the unnecessary escalation of healthcare costs. This additional niacinamide would probably nearly return the daily dietary intake to that experienced centuries ago before the advent of widespread artificial fertilizer use and food processing.

This public health strategy would not be new. During the Second World War, the United States government mandated the enrichment of flour with niacinamide. However, current dietary levels are still too low. Increasing the intake of niacinamide would carry no known risks, since it is not addictive, nor is it a narcotic, euphoriant, or analgesic. In short, a small investment in niacinamide would provide huge economic and social benefits to society with no known associated risks. Still, some people would require far more vitamin B-3 than others, either because of pre-existing diseases and disorders or as a result of their genetic inheritance.

The Case of Sickle Cell Anemia

The question remains, "Why would a genetic aberration that lowers niacin production in the body and results in so many diseases or disorders become so widespread among the human population?" Perhaps the answer can be obtained by studying sickle cell anemia. Roughly one out of every 400 Afro-Americans develops sickle cell anemia. In those with this chronic hereditary disease, many of their red blood cells form rigid crescent or sickle shapes that cannot pass through capillaries. Affected children often die during adolescence of strokes, heart disease, and infections. Sickle cell anemia also causes sufferers painful, unpredictable health crises. Those children who survive are underweight and slow to mature.[5] How is it that a genetic, highly damaging disease can be so widespread amongst the Afro-American population in the USA? What's in it for Darwin? Or more correctly asked, what is the evolutionary advantage that this mutation gives to Afro-Americans that makes its obvious disadvantages worthwhile? After all, as McElroy and Townsend point out, "It is only the phenotypic characteristics that give some advantage of degree of Darwinian fitness that are subject to selective action."[6]

At first glance, the sickle cell anemia trait appears to provide Afro-Americans with the very reverse of Darwinian fitness. After all, those with this genetic disorder tend to die in adolescence. Even if they don't, they are usually underweight, slow to develop, and often sick. These are not the type of people who might be anticipated to have larger families than the norm and so have a disproportionate effect on the human gene pool.

As anticipated, the differential reproduction and mortality linked to this genotype in the United States are both negative: sufferers reproduce less and die younger. One might expect that, as a result, over time the mutation responsible for sickle cell anemia would have disappeared. This has not been the case. Why? Malaria has plagued humanity for thousands of years.[7] Even now it affects an estimated 200 million people every year, causing some 2 million deaths. In tropical Africa, for example, it kills about 1 million people annually, most of those being children.[8] The disease also contributes to death from other causes, including pneumonia, anemia, and kidney failure. The anemia associated with malaria is linked to miscarriage, still-birth, and low birth weight.[10]

Malaria is caused by a protozoan parasite of the genus *Plasmodium*, which infects red blood cells. The protozoans cannot live outside their hosts and depend completely on the glucose, enzymes, and metabolism of such cells to survive.[11] This parasitic relationship eventually destroys the red blood cells, usually at 2- or 3-day intervals. The release of associated waste products and pigments causes the intermittent fever and chills seen in malaria sufferers. *Plasmodium* protozoa are spread from one human to another by four species of mosquitoes.

At some time in the past, a point mutation occurred in one of the human DNA base pair codes for the hemoglobin protein chains.[12, 13] Instead of glutamic acid at the sixth position, as is usually the case, valine was produced. This substitution affected hemoglobin's level of oxygen affinity and led to the distortion of the cell membrane into an irregular, sickled shape. *Plasmodium* do not appreciate this abnormality. As a result, people with this sickling trait are unlikely to suffer as much from malaria. They are not completely immune, but, if infected, the disease is less severe.

In heterozygotes, who usually do not exceed 30% to 40% of the population living in areas where malaria is commonplace, the sickling trait provides both normal and abnormal hemoglobin in every blood cell. This is a characteristic that increases their chances of surviving malaria to reproduce.[14] In those who are homozygous for sickle cell anemia, this characteristic still helps to resist malaria, but their cells have nothing but abnormal hemoglobin. As a consequence, they develop sickle cell anemia, which, as described, is often fatal.

The offspring of two parents who carry the trait (heterozygotes) have a 25% percent chance of being born with sickle cell anemia (homozygotes).[15] In West African populations, this occurs in roughly 4% of children, most of whom die before they can reproduce. The sickle cell trait has survived in Afro-Americans because, despite the high toll sickle cell anemia takes, the trait is counterbalanced by the benefits of reduced susceptibility to malaria that it provides. This is called a balanced polymorphism.

Interestingly, in regions where malaria has been wiped out and where the sickling trait only brings disadvantages, its prevalence begins to decline. In the United States, for example, it is now found in only 8.5% of Afro-Americans. As a result, sickle cell anemia occurs in a fraction of 1% of this population,[16] causing roughly 350 deaths annually.[17]

This brings us back to diseases associated with niacin deficiency. There are numerous, extremely dangerous diseases and disorders associated with our inability to synthesize adequate vitamin B-3. Any genetic aberration promoting such a deficiency state, if it was to diffuse widely in the human population, must have carried with it some enormous counterbalancing advantage. If it did not, it would soon have disappeared from the human gene pool. What, then, are the advantages of the apparent inadequate synthesis of niacin?

Adrenochrome Trade-Off

Since high levels of niacin are so beneficial, how could it be advantageous to lose most of our ability to synthesize it? One possible answer to this question is that vitamin B-3 may be highly antagonistic with some other substance that also carries major health benefits. If this is the case, a balanced genetic polymorphism might permit humanity to gain some of the advantages of both niacin and this antagonist. This was, apparently, the case. The antagonist(s) of niacin involved in this trade-off were adrenochrome and its derivatives.

Stress

Stress is the easiest way to promote the metabolism of adrenaline in the human body. Although medical interest in stress can be traced back to Hippocrates,[18] it was not until the 1920s that psychologist Walter Cannon confirmed that response to stress is part of a unified mind-body system.[19] Cannon was able to show that various stressors, including extreme cold, lack of oxygen, and emotion-arousing incidents trigger an outpouring of epinephrine (adrenaline) and norepinephrine (noradrenaline). These enter the bloodstream from sympathetic nerve endings in the inner adrenal glands.[20]

In those stressed, the sympathetic nervous system increases respiration and heart rate, diverts blood to skeletal muscles, and releases fat from storage. All these changes prepare the body for what Cannon called "fight or flight" and are obviously part of a response system that has evolved in an effort to deal with perceived threats. In any biochemical evolutionary trade-off, the ability to escape from life-threatening hazards would have to rank very highly.

Unfortunately, in situations of chronic stress, the fight or flight response becomes counterproductive, leading to a cumulative build up of adrenaline, noradrenaline, and cortisol. If these substances are not properly metabolized, long-term stress appears to promote disorders ranging from headaches and high blood pressure to rheumatoid arthritis and allergies.[21] What is significant here is that the fight or flight response to stress is associated with an elevation of adrenaline, whose oxidation can lead to an excess of adrenochrome. Perhaps it is not surprising, then, that chronic stress is often linked to anxiety, poor concentration, depression, anger, frustration, fear, and sadness.[22] If the individual being stressed carries one of the genetic aberrations linked to schizophrenia, adrenochrome levels are likely to be higher than normal and may be linked to paranoia and hallucinations that this indole causes when taken accidentally or experimentally.[23]

Intelligence and Creativity

Besides being a hallucinogen, adrenochrome is a highly reactive neurotoxin that, in schizophrenia, undermines at least three major biochemical systems. It is an antagonist of the hormone triiodothyronine and can damage the thyroid. In chronic schizophrenics, this gland impairment appears permanent. Adrenochrome also has a Jekyll and Hyde relationship with serotonin and, so, impacts on tryptophan and its other chief metabolite, niacin. At low levels, serotonin appears to stimulate adrenochrome formation, while at higher levels it retards the process. Adrenochrome also generates numerous free radicals, causing oxidative stress, eventually exhausting the schizophrenic antioxidant defense systems, creating deficiencies of glutathione peroxidase, superoxide dismutase, and catalase. Complicating the impacts of high adrenochrome conversion from adrenaline are the numerous interactions that normally occur between tri-iodothyronine, serotonin, and the three major components of the antioxidant defense system.[24]

In the early 1950s, Dr Hoffer and Dr Osmond showed that the production of adrenochrome could be reduced by high doses of niacin. During times of stress, noradrenaline is converted to adrenaline and then to adrenochrome. Hoffer and his coworkers knew the conversion of noradrenalin to adrenaline requires methyl groups, which are provided by methyl donors.[25] Noradrenalin is a methyl acceptor that adds one methyl group to become adrenaline. They argued that if they could prevent the addition of this methyl group to noradrenaline, there should be a corresponding reduction in the amount of adrenaline available for conversion to adrenochrome.

Accordingly, they decided to use high doses of niacin, another natural methyl acceptor, to reduce the conversion rate of noradrenaline to adrenaline and then to adrenochrome. Double-blind controlled experiments conducted on acute schizophrenics with high doses of niacin (usually 3 to 6 g daily) were very successful, outperforming the then conventional treatments and reducing suicide rates.[26]

Niacin can lower the body's production of adrenochrome and its derivatives. Conversely, high levels of adrenochrome can also reduce the availability of niacin for other uses in the body beyond reducing the availability of adrenaline. There could, therefore, be a genetically balanced polymorphism if adrenochrome and its derivatives had benefits comparable to those of niacin.

The balanced morphism idea has reappeared in the medical literature at various times. Dr Hoffer, for example, has argued that the family members if schizophrenics who do not develop the disease tend to be unusually intelligent.[27] This concept underlies Dr David Horrobin's book, *The Madness of Adam and Eve,* in which he argues: "Schizophrenia can affect people of all abilities in all strata of society, but it does with surprising frequency seem to affect the families of the great, the good, the clever, the rich, the ambitious, the intellectual and the creative. ... The genes for schizophrenia, which are likely to include genes for bipolar disorder, dyslexia, high intelligence and schizotypy, are responsible for most of the religious sense, most of the technical and artistic creativity, and most of the leadership qualities in modern humans."[28] Of course, it is these genes which, in schizophrenics, promote overexposure to adrenochrome.

This belief is not new. Galton's eugenic ideas, involving the selective 'weeding out' of schizophrenics and their families, were rejected by Henry Maudsley, the greatest psychiatrist in London in the second half of the 19th century, because he knew that schizophrenia occurred repeatedly in the great families of Victorian Britain.[29] Maudsley recognized that an eugenic program, designed to eliminate schizophrenia, would inevitably prevent the birth of some of Britain's future most creative and dynamic individuals. Myerson and Boyl came to the same conclusion in the United States, where they found that American presidents, philosophers, writers, scientists, and physicians all had schizophrenic relatives who had been treated at McLean Hospital, near Boston.[30] A recent Scandinavian study has established that children of university graduates are almost twice as likely to develop schizophrenia than the children of non-graduates.[31] Another study has shown that Icelandic males, with psychotic family members, seem to have more skills and abilities and contain higher achievers in a variety of fields than do those with families without those who have this illness.[32] Healthy relatives of psychotic patients, for example, publish more books of fiction and poetry and perform better in school, particularly in mathematics.[33]

Cancer Prevention

As early as 1893, H. Snow argued that psychiatric patients were immune to cancer.[34] His view was supported in 1909 by the Commissioners in Lunacy for England and Wales, who reported that their mentally unbalanced charges seemed to be relatively cancer-free.[35] Since then, numerous studies have shown that although psychiatric patients experience higher general mortality levels than the general public from a wide variety causes, cancer is an exception to this rule.[36] Although some researchers have been unable to discover statistically significant negative correlations between schizophrenia and cancer,[37, 38] several others have confirmed a lower than normal cancer incidence in psychiatric patients.[39-41]

D. Rice, for example, in 1979, claimed bronchogenic carcinoma had never been recorded in a chronic schizophrenic in-patient, despite the fact that the great majority of them smoked cigarettes.[42] Craig and Lin supported Rice's position and also documented lower than normal lung cancer incidence in such in-patients.[43]

Several more very large scale examinations of the schizophrenia-cancer relationship have been carried out in the past 20 years. W. Gulbinat and coworkers, for example, studied the incidence of cancer among schizophrenics in Nagasaki, Japan, Aarhus, Denmark, and Honolulu, Hawaii, and compared these rates with that of the local general public.[44] Interestingly, although cancer incidence was generally much lower among Caucasian schizophrenics, it was elevated in Japanese schizophrenics in both Hawaii and Japan. Of particular interest here were the very low relative risks of lung cancer in both Danish males (rr = 0.38) and females (rr = 0.33) during the period 1957 to 1980.

D. Lichtermann and colleagues also conducted a study in Finland that followed up the subsequent health of 26,996 patients treated for schizophrenia in the period 1969 to 1991.[45] The aim of this research was to establish which of these patients had developed cancer, during the time period 1971 to 1996. They could determine this by linking schizophrenic patients' records with the Finnish Cancer Registry. These researchers deduced that, because of their excessive smoking, there was a relative increase in cancer risk in schizophrenics, but there was a consistently lower than normal incidence of cancer in their parents and siblings.

M. Cohen and coworkers used data from the US 1986 National Mortality Followback Survey (which examined 1% of all USA deaths in that year, in detail), death certificates, hospital records, and interviews with informants and decedents' families to study the schizophrenia-cancer association.[46] They discovered that the unadjusted odds ratio for cancer among schizophrenics, in the United States, was only 0.62. After controlling for race, gender, age, education, marital status, net worth, smoking, and hospitalization in the year before death, this odds ratio fell to 0.59 (95% CI 0.38-0.93). Cohen and colleagues concluded that, in the United States, there was much less risk of a schizophrenic developing cancer than a member of the general public suffering this diagnosis. This also appeared to be true of the immediate families of schizophrenics.[47]

This conclusion seems to be consistent with Dr Hoffer's experience. He has treated some 800 patients diagnosed with a wide spectrum of cancer. Only five of these were schizophrenic. Three suffered from breast cancer, one cancer of the thyroid, and the fifth patient had lymphoma. Every case was responsive to treatment, with an average survival time of 10 years. Hoffer also has treated approximately 5,000 schizophrenics since 1952, about 500 of whom are still current patients. Only 0.1%, the five previously described, also have had cancer.[48-50]

Lower cancer incidence has been recorded among schizophrenics treated by both conventional physicians and orthomolecular doctors. Since the former use drugs and the latter vitamins and minerals, it follows that the depressed cancer incidence must be related to the biochemistry of schizophrenia itself. Taken as a whole, the available evidence seems to show that schizophrenics, as well as their siblings and parents, are less susceptible to cancer than the general public. These conclusions appear to be compatible with one or more genetic risk factors for schizophrenia that provide a selective advantage against cancer. Many of the genetic aberrations that promote schizophrenia, but protect against cancer, are apparently involved in the metabolism of adrenochrome and its derivatives.[51, 52]

If this is true, then adrenochrome and associated catecholamine o-quinones should be protective against many types of cancer. There is growing evidence that this is, indeed, the case. As early as 1970, K. Yamafuji and coworkers argued that noradrenaline or adrenaline had antitumor properties.[53] However, the evidence strongly suggests that it is not adrenaline, but its oxidation product(s) adrenochrome or derivative(s) that are most likely to protect against cancer. Fortunately, there is experimental evidence to support this possibility. Matrix Pharmaceuticals has a US patent for an IntraDose Injectable Gel that contains cisplatin and epinephrine (adrenaline).[54] This gel is designed for direct injection into tumors. Interestingly, cisplatin is a very strong oxidant which must rapidly convert the adrenaline to adrenochrome. While Matrix Pharmaceuticals argue that cisplatin is the active cytotoxic (cancer destroying) agent in IntraDose, it seems much more probable that adrenochrome and its derivatives are more effective in killing cancer cells.

IntraDose is undergoing a series of Phase III open-label clinical studies, in which it is injected into patients' most troublesome tumors. The results have been very impressive. To illustrate, in women with advanced breast cancer, 14 out of 30 tumors, that is 47%, were reduced by 50% or more in volume for at least 28 days after IntraDose treatment. In five cases, tumors completely disappeared, while eight others were reduced in volume by over 80%.[55] Results also were very good in malignant melanoma patients. Eleven of the 25 most troublesome tumors were at least halved in volume, while four disappeared completely.[56] IntraDose also proved very beneficial in the treatment of esophageal cancer,[57] cancer of the liver,[58] and cancers of the head and neck.[59]

The evidence is good, therefore, that adrenochrome and its derivative(s) not only promote intelligence and creativity, but also protect against a wide range of cancers.

Benefits of Vitamin B-3 Therapy

Humanity has virtually lost the ability to synthesize niacin. This probably had relatively little negative consequence when diets were high in this vitamin, but mineral-deficient fertilizers and food processing are depleting diets of a wide range of essential nutrients, including vitamin B-3. As a consequence, the numerous niacin deficiency diseases, including arthritis, heart diseases, and schizophrenia, are becoming much more prevalent.

There have, however, been advantages associated with this loss of the ability to synthesize niacin. This vitamin is an antagonist of adrenochrome and its derivatives, which appear to promote intelligence and creativity and reduce susceptibility to cancer. There seems, therefore, to be a balanced polymorphism at work, ensuring that genetically the benefits and costs of a decreased ability to metabolize niacin are offset against those associated with high levels of adrenochrome and its associated derivatives.

Ideally, then, we should attempt to obtain the benefits of both niacin and adrenochrome without the disadvantages of either. On the one hand, niacin deficiency can be easily overcome by supplementation, usually combined with high dose vitamin C. Elevated adrenochrome is a double-edged sword. It appears to promote both intelligence and psychosis, while protecting against cancer. As seen in the treatment of schizophrenics, where excessively elevated levels of adrenochrome cause psychosis, they must be lowered by natural methyl acceptors, such as niacin and coenzyme

Q10. However, the successful treatment of cancer may require deliberately stimulating adrenochrome levels to the point at which they cause temporary psychosis.

As a species, we need to be smart enough to manipulate the body levels of niacin and adrenochrome and its derivatives so that we can gain their benefits without paying the health costs of shortages of either.

References

[1] Pauling L. Orthomolecular psychiatry. Science 1968;160:265-271.

[2] Pauling L. Evolution and the need for ascorbic acid. Proceedings of the National Academy of Sciences 1970;67:1643-48.

[3] Stone I. The Healing Factor: "Vitamin C" Against Disease. New York NY: Grosset & Dunlap, 1977.

[4] Niacin. http://pune.sancharnet.in/spr_keshri/b3.htm

[5] Pearson HA. Sickle cell anaemia: Clinical management during the early years of life. In: Abramson H, Bertles JF, Wethers DL (eds.). Sickle Cell Disease. St. Louis, MO: CV Mosby, 1973:244-51.

[6] McElroy A, and Townsend PK. Medical Anthropology in Ecological Perspectives. Boulder, CO: Westview Press, 1989.

[7] McElroy A, and Townsend PK. Medical Anthropology in Ecological Perspectives. Boulder, CO: Westview Press, 1989.

[8] McFalls JA Jr., McFalls MH. Disease and Fertility. New York, NY: Academic Press, 1982.

[10] McFalls JA Jr., McFalls MH. Disease and Fertility. New York, NY: Academic Press, 1982.

[11] McElroy A, and Townsend PK. Medical Anthropology in Ecological Perspectives. Boulder, CO: Westview Press, 1989.

[12] McElroy A, and Townsend PK. Medical Anthropology in Ecological Perspectives. Boulder, CO: Westview Press, 1989.

[13] Stini W. Ecology and Human Adaptation. Dubuque, IA: Wm C Brown, 1975.

[14] McElroy A, and Townsend PK. Medical Anthropology in Ecological Perspectives. Boulder, CO: Westview Press, 1989.

[15] Fishbein's Illustrated Medical and Health Encyclopedia. Westport, CT: HS Stuttman, 1985;4:1305-09.

[16] Johnson MI. The world and the sickle-cell gene. New York, NY: TradoMedic Books, 1984.

[17] Gary LE. (1977). The sickle-cell controversy. In: AS Baer (ed.). Heredity and Society: Readings in Social Genetics. New York: Macmillan, 1977:361-73.

[18] Myers DG. Psychology. New York, NY: Worth Publishers, 1992.

[19] Myers DG. Psychology. New York, NY: Worth Publishers, 1992.

[20] Myers DG. Psychology. New York, NY: Worth Publishers, 1992.

[21] Mind/Body Education Center. The Fight or Flight Response. http://www.mindbodymed.com/EducationCenter/fight.html

[22] Mind/Body Education Center. The Fight or Flight Response. http://www.mindbodymed.com/EducationCenter/fight.html

[23] Dishinger RC. Bad behavior and illness are caused by biochemical imbalances. Owensboro, KT: Medici Music Press, 1998.

[24] Foster HD. What Really Causes Schizophrenia. Victoria, BC: Trafford Publishing, 2003.

[25] Hoffer A. Vitamin B-3 and Schizophrenia: Discovery, Recovery, Controversy. Kingston, ON: Quarry Health Books, 1998.

[26] Hoffer A. Vitamin B-3 and Schizophrenia: Discovery, Recovery, Controversy. Kingston, ON: Quarry Health Books, 1998.

[27] Hoffer A. Vitamin B-3 and Schizophrenia: Discovery, Recovery, Controversy. Kingston, ON: Quarry Health Books, 1998.

[28] Horrobin D. The Madness of Adam and Eve. London, UK: Transworld Publishers, 2002.

[29] Horrobin D. The Madness of Adam and Eve. London, UK: Transworld Publishers, 2002.

[30] Horrobin D. The Madness of Adam and Eve. London, UK: Transworld Publishers, 2002.

[31] Karlsson JL. Relation of mathematical ability to psychosis in Iceland. Clinical Genetics 1999;56(6):447-49.

[32] Karlsson JL. Relation of mathematical ability to psychosis in Iceland. Clinical Genetics 1999;56(6):447-49.

[33] Horrobin D. The Madness of Adam and Eve. London, UK: Transworld Publishers, 2002.

[34] Snow H. A treatise: Practical and theoretic on cancers and the cancer process. London, UK: Churchill, 1893.

[35] Gottesman II. Schizophrenia Genesis: The Origins of Madness. New York, NY: W.H. Freeman, 1991:187.

[36] Gulbinat W, Dupoint A, Jablensky A, Jensen OM, Marsella A, Nakane Y, et al. Cancer incidence of schizophrenic patients. Results of record linkage studies in three countries. Brit J Psychiat 1992;161:(Suppl 18):75-85.

[37] Innes G, Millar WM. Mortality among psychiatric patients. Scott Med J 1970;15:142-49.

[38] Odegaard O. The excess mortality of the insane. Acta Psychiat Scand 1952;27:353-67.

[39] Peller S, Stephenson CS. Cancer in the mentally ill. Public Health Rep 1941;56:132-49.

[41] Cohen M, Dembling B, Schorling J. The association between schizophrenias and cancer: A population-based mortality study. Schizophrenia Res 2002;57(2-3):139-46.

[42] Rice D. No lung cancer in schizophrenics. Brit J Psychiat 1979;134:128.

[43] Craig TJ, Lin SP. Cancer and mental illness. Compr psychiat 1981;22:404-10.

[44] Gulbinat W, Dupoint A, Jablensky A, Jensen OM, Marsella A, Nakane Y, et al. Cancer incidence of schizophrenic patients. Results of record linkage studies in three countries. Brit J Psychiat 1992;161:(Suppl 18):75-85.

[45] Lichtermann D, Ekelund J, Pukkala E, Tanskanen A, Lonnquist J. Incidence of cancer among persons with schizophrenia and their relatives. Arch Gen Psychiat 2001;58(6):573-78.

[46] Cohen M, Dembling B, Schorling J. The association between schizophrenias and cancer: A population-based mortality study. Schizophrenia Res 2002;57 (2-3):139-46.

[47] Lichtermann D, Ekelund J, Pukkala E, Tanskanen A, Lonnquist J. Incidence of cancer among persons with schizophrenia and their relatives. Arch Gen Psychiat 2001;58(6):573-78.

[48] Hoffer A. Vitamin B-3 and Schizophrenia: Discovery, Recovery, Controversy. Kingston, ON: Quarry Health Books, 1998.

[50] Foster HD, Hoffer A. Schizophrenia and cancer: The adrenochrome balanced morphism. Medical Hypotheses 2004;62:415-19.

[51] Hoffer A. Vitamin B-3 and Schizophrenia: Discovery, Recovery, Controversy. Kingston, ON: Quarry Health Books, 1998.

[52] Foster HD. What Really Causes Schizophrenia. Victoria, BC: Trafford Publishing, 2003.

[53] Yamafuji K, Murakami H, Shinozuka M. Antitumor activity of dopa, dopamine, noradrenaline or adrenalin and their reaction with nucleic acids. Z Krebsforsch Klin Onkol 1970;73(3):195-203.

[54] Pharmalicensing. Matrix receives IntraDose patent June 24, 2000. Available from: http://www.docguide.com/dg.nsf/PrintPrint/69A02FE8488ACBDD85256690004 9EF6B.

[55] Doctor's guide to medical and other news. October 1, 1998. IntraDose shows good response rate in most troublesome breast cancer tumors. Available from: http://www.docguide.com/dg.nsf/PrintPrint/69A02FE8488ACBDD85256690004 9EF6B.

[56] Doctor's guide to medical and other news. November 13, 1998. IntraDose shows encouraging results for malignant melanoma and breast cancer. Available from: http://www.docguide.com/dg.nsf/PrintPrint/3C50DF24B0822F4E852566BB006E 290C.

[57] Business Wire. September 15, 1999. Matrix IntraDose injectable gel featured in four presentations at the annual meeting of the European Cancer Congress. Available from: http://www.slip.net/-mcdavis/databas2/gel_4.htm.

[58] Doctor's guide global edition. November 4, 1999. CFS meeting: IntraDose shows promise in treatment of primary liver cancer. Available from: http://www.pslgroup.com/dg/1424a6.htm.

[59] OBGYN.net e-mail Newsletter. December 17, 2001. Matrix submits European application for IntraDose approval. Head and Neck Cancer. Available from: http://www.obgyn.net/newsrx/general_health-Head_And_Neck_Cancer-20011217-9.asp.

Vitamin B-3
Responsive Diseases
and Conditions

PELLAGRA

Prevalence

Classical Pellagra

Pellagra was known in Europe for near 200 years before being diagnosed in the United States, where it was first identified in 1902. It was initially described by Don Gasper Casal, a physician in the Spanish court. In 1735 Casal noted the illness among poor peasants and called it "mal de la rosa" because all affected patients had a typical reddish glossy rash on their hands and feet.[1]

In the early 20th century, patients suffering from pellagra filled one-third of mental hospitals in the southeastern United States.[2] It is estimated that between 1906 and 1940, three million Americans developed pellagra and 100,000 of these died from it. Pellagra was particularly common amongst the Southern poor, who ate meals that were typically dominated by meat (pork fatback), molasses, and cornmeal. Pellagra is still a significant problem in those areas of the developing world, where white rice or maize dominate diets. According to M.C. Latham, the highest recorded recent prevalence has occurred in the 1990s in South Africa.[3] Some 50% of patients seen in a clinic in Transvaal showed evidence of pellagra, while the majority of adults in a Pretoria mental hospital suffered from this disorder.

In 1914, Dr Joseph Goldberg was assigned by the United States Public Health Service to identify the cause of the pellagra epidemic in the Southern states.[4, 5] He soon discovered that the well-fed staff of both mental hospitals and prisons did not develop pellagra, while malnourished patients and inmates often did. He concluded that pellagra must be a nutritional illness, not one caused by germs, as was generally believed. To prove the validity of his hypothesis, Goldberg and his assistants and even his wife held "filth parties," at which they injected themselves with the blood of pellagra patients. Goldberg and supporters also ingested patients' scabs, feces, and body fluids, but did not develop pellagra as a consequence. In addition, in exchange for full pardons, a group of Mississippi prison inmates volunteered to eat very poor quality diets. Within a few months, many developed pellagra. When fresh vegetables, milk, and meat were added to their diets, all symptoms of pellagra quickly reversed.

Although Goldberg had clearly shown that pellagra was a nutritional deficiency disease that could be prevented and cured by changes in diet, it was not until 1937 that researchers at the University of Wisconsin discovered the key vitamin involved was niacin.[6] Interestingly, early pellagrologists found that long-term classical pellagra had to be treated with up to 600 mg of vitamin B-3 daily. In contrast only 10 mg of niacin were needed to prevent the illness. That is, the low dosages, suggested by the vitamins-as-prevention paradigm, were adequate to stop the disease developing in healthy individuals, but were totally inadequate to cure the illness in long-term patients, who needed the high vitamins-as-drugs paradigm dosages. High doses of vitamin B-3 soon emptied developed world mental hospitals of their pellagrins.

Subclinical Pellagra

There is also clear evidence of widespread subclinical pellagra in the general population. Subclinical pellagra has, in fact, become pandemic. Approximately 50% of the North American population, it is estimated, will be responsive to increased doses of vitamin B-3, no matter what their symptoms and signs. The great majority of patients with schizophrenia, arthritis, addictions, cancer, cardiovascular disease, stress-related anxiety and fatigue, as well as other diseases and conditions described in this book, are suffering from subclinical pellagra. All patients with diseases that respond to supplements of vitamin B-3 are suffering from subclinical pellagra. The main difference between classical pellagra and subclinical pellagra is that subclinical pellagrins do not have the skin lesions typical of classical pellagrins. While small doses of vitamin B-3 are effective in treating non-chronic pellagra, a vitamin B-3 deficiency disorder, much larger doses are needed to treat chronic pellagra, a vitamin dependency disease.

Role of Vitamin B-3

Classical Pellagra

Pellagra was the first health condition to be treated successfully with vitamin B-3. With this discovery, classical pellagra, characterized by the four 'Ds' – diarrhea, dermatitis, dementia, and death – almost disappeared in North America. In the United States during the 1940s, vitamin B-3 (niacinamide) was added to flour by decree of public health agencies, although in Canada, flour enrichment was not permitted for several years because it was considered an adulteration of food. [7] Nevertheless, the Director of the Department of Indian Affairs insisted that flour sold to Canada's aboriginal people must be niacinamide enriched. Overseas during the Second World War, Canadian armed forces were often "forced" to eat adulterated American bread containing niacinamide.

Even with the widespread supplementation of niacinamide in flour, classical pellagra has not entirely disappeared. Dr Hoffer has seen one case during his 50 years in practice. The face, neck, and shoulders of the patient were covered with a peculiar symmetrical brownish discoloration. The patient reported that she had suffered from this condition for many years, consulting 12 different doctors, many of them dermatologists. Of the 12, one suggested that she keep out of the sun, not recognizing that she had pellagra. She recovered soon after beginning to take large doses of vitamin B-3.

Subclinical Pellagra

The early pellagrologists in the 1930s recognized widespread subclinical pellagra, which manifests in a wide variety of symptoms. As Tom Spies and his colleagues noted in 1938: "Subclinical pellagrins are noted for the multiplicity of their complaints, among which are many that are usually classed as neurasthenic. The most common of these symptoms are fatigue, insomnia, anorexia, vertigo, burning sensation in various parts of the body, numbness, palpitations, nervousness, a feeling of unrest and anxiety, headache, forgetfulness, apprehension, and distractibility. The conduct of a pellagrins may be normal, but he feels incapable of mental or physical effort, even though he may be ambulatory."[8] To control the symptoms of subclinical pellagra that had been present for a long time required up to 600 mg of vitamin B-3 daily. At the time, this was considered an enormous dose when only 10 mg per needed to prevent classical pellagra.

Clinical Evidence

Pellagra and Schizophrenia

Clinically, pellagrins and schizophrenics are the same. Although schizophrenic patients do not suffer as much as pellagrins from diarrhea, dermatitis, dementia, and death, these conditions are so alike that they cannot be easily distinguished and are, almost certainly, part of the same syndrome.

Before the introduction of pure vitamin B-3, the diagnostic differentiation between pellagra and schizophrenia was based on the history and economic status of the patients. If they were poor, lived on a very rich corn-based diet, and consumed little protein, they were called pellagrins. Otherwise, these patients were called schizophrenics.

After vitamin B-3 became widely available, if patients responded very quickly to niacin treatment, in a matter of weeks, they were diagnosed as having pellagra. If they did not respond rapidly, they were classified as schizophrenics. For example, Dr V. L. Evans describes a patient who had been ill for 11 years and was clearly psychotic, but when given 500 mg of nicotinic acid, she became normal in only 4 days. "If it had not been for her response to nicotinic acid therapy," he explained, "the case would probably have been classified as schizophrenic or toxic psychosis."[9] Today, pellagra is typically seen as a vitamin B-3 deficiency disease, while schizophrenia is a vitamin B-3 dependency disease because patients need much more vitamin B-3 than the average population.

Dr G. Green, a general practitioner, reported that he saw 183 subclinical pellagrins, 9 of whom were likely schizophrenic, in 2 years, amongst the First Nations population around Prince Albert in Saskatchewan.[10] In his report on the situation he concluded: "The clinical proof of the condition is the prompt disappearance of the symptom complex after the administration of large doses of niacin or niacinamide. I have been using 1.5 to 6 grams a day with excellent results."

Pellagrins are also typically deficient in protein, tryptophan, other vitamins, and essential fatty acids.

Children's Attention and Behavior Disorders

Today, children with subclinical pellagra, as it was described in the 1930s, are classified in the *American Psychiatric Association Diagnostic Manual* as suffering from one of the attention deficit disorders, such as ADHD (attention deficit hyperactivity disorder), commonly treated with the popular drug Ritalin.

In his book *Healing Children's Attention and Behavior Disorders*, Dr Hoffer has shown these conditions can be treated effectively with orthomolecular medicine.[11] As with the treatment of other syndromes, large doses of vitamin B-3 and other nutrients, such as vitamin C, are used, with consideration given to possible allergies, especially to milk and sugar. Medication is prescribed if needed, but this is very rarely necessary.

Dr Hoffer has treated approximately 2,000 children under the age of 14 since 1960 for attention and behavior disorders.[12] More than 90% of these patients have responded to orthomolecular treatment with full or nearly full recoveries. None of these children was ever started on Ritalin or other drugs, and, in most cases, when the children were taking this drug, they were able to substitute vitamins. The results have been, and continue to be, very good. Vitamin B-3 is one of the most important nutrients for most childhood health conditions, except for children with infantile autism, where pyridoxine is more useful.

References

[1] Rajakumar K. Pellagra in the United States: A historical perspective. Southern Medical Journal 2000;93(3):272-277.

[2] Rajakumar K. Pellagra in the United States: A historical perspective. Southern Medical Journal 2000;93(3):272-277.

[3] Latham MC. Human nutrition in the Developing World. FAO Food & Nutrition Series No. 29. Rome: Food & Agricultural Organizations of the United Nations, 1997.

[4] Goldberg J. The etiology of pellagra: The significance of certain epidemiological observations with respect thereto. Public Health Rep. 1914; 29:1683-1686.

[5] Goldberg J, Wheeler GA. Experimental pellagra: A test of diet among institutional inmates. Public Health Rep. 1915;30:3117-3131.

[6] Elvehjem CA, Madden RJ, Strong FM et al. Relation of nicotinic acid and nicotinic acid amide to canine black tongue. J Am Chem Soc 1937;59:1767-1768.

[7] Wilder RM. A brief history of the enrichment of bread and flour. JAMA 1956;162:1539-1541.

[8] Spies TD, Aring CD, Gelperin J, Bean BW. The mental symptoms of pellagra. Am J Med Science 1938;196:461.

[9] Evans VL. Pellagra with psychosis and minimal symptoms. JAMA 1939;112:1249-1250.

[10] Green G. Subclinical pellagra. In: Orthomolecular Psychiatry: Treatment of Schizophrenia. Hawkins D, Pauling L (eds.). San Francisco, CA: WH Freeman & Co., 1973:411-33.

[11] Hoffer A. Hoffer's A.B.C. of Natural Nutrition for Children. Kingston, ON: Quarry Health Books, 1999; revised as Healing Children's Attention and Behavior Disorders, Toronto ON: CCNM Press, 2004.

[12] Hoffer A. Hoffer's A.B.C. of Natural Nutrition for Children. Kingston, ON: Quarry Health Books,1999; revised as Healing Children's Attention and Behavior Disorders. Toronto ON: CCNM Press, 2004.

SCHIZOPHRENIA SYNDROME

Prevalence

S chizophrenia is a relatively common disorder. In North America, 1% to 2% of the population will have at least one schizophrenic episode during their lifetime. The lower figure of 1% is usually quoted, but the higher figure of 2% is more likely to be correct. There is no doubt that many patients have some of the manifestations of schizophrenia, but because they have not developed hallucinations and delusions, they will not be diagnosed as schizophrenic.

In Canada, schizophrenics have the second highest number of hospitalizations among the various other mental illnesses. About 300,000 people are currently sick with the disorder.[1] In the United States, approximately 2.7 million Americans suffer from schizophrenia.[2]

The total cost to society of each schizophrenic patient, whether untreated or given drugs, is roughly $2 million dollars over the lifespan of their illness. This figure includes expenditures on medication, hospitalization, welfare, police, and court costs, as well as loss of productivity. Medication expenses may be as high as $5,000 per year. Each day a schizophrenic spends in hospital costs more than $1,200. Court and legal costs are unknown, but in Victoria, British Columbia, for example, the local police are called about 300 times each year to deal with chronic, homeless, schizophrenic patients. Beyond this, given that healthy, normal people in North America have an average income of roughly $40,000 annually and pay income tax of about $8,000, the loss of society per schizophrenic in tax is roughly $300,000 during the 40-year life span of their illness. Fortunately, many of these costs can be eliminated with the use of vitamin B-3 to treat schizophrenia, not to mention the human toll in suffering and suicide among schizophrenia patients and their families.

Role of Vitamin B-3

Schizophrenia is not a homogeneous condition. Rather, it is a syndrome caused by a number of factors that appear unrelated. This was recognized more than 100 years ago. In the old textbooks, the differential diagnosis included dementia praecox (now called schizophrenia); general paresis of the insane (caused by the syphilis spirochete); scurvy (due to a deficiency of ascorbic acid); and pellagra (caused by vitamin B-3 deficiency). In his classic book on *Dementia Praecox,* Dr E. Bleuler subdivided this condition into such categories as paranoid or catatonic, based on the clinical expression of the syndrome. More recently, Dr Carl C. Pfeiffer divided schizophrenic patients into three major groups: the first excrete kryptopyrrole in their urine (pyroluria); the second have elevated blood histamine; the third have low blood histamine.

Such clinical states are really syndromes, not diseases. They only become a diagnosed disease when the cause has been identified. Dr Pfeiffer recognized more than 25 different potential causal factors or, to use Professor Harold Foster's terminology, triggers. Knowing that schizophrenia is a syndrome with many causal factors forces diagnosticians to search for such triggers and to treat the basic biochemical pathologic end-reactions that produce the characteristic schizophrenic syndrome. In the same way, severe chest pain that is worse with breathing, high fever, and a cough probably means pneumonia, but until the necessary laboratory tests are completed, it cannot be known if these symptoms are caused by the pneumococcus bacteria, a virus, cancer, or tuberculosis.

Among these various triggers for schizophrenia, two emerge as major causes: reactions to food and other allergens; and vitamin B-3 deficiency and dependency. Other common triggers include pyridoxine deficiency and hypothyroidism. Less common causes include scurvy, hallucinogenic experiences (from LSD and mescaline), drug toxicities (such as atropine and amphetamines), copper excess, and zinc deficiency. Only schizophrenia caused by a lack of vitamin B-3 will be discussed here.

Clinical Evidence

In his book *Vitamin B-3 and Schizophrenia: Discovery, Recovery, Controversy*, Dr Hoffer reviews the development of clinical research in this field, while in his book *Healing Schizophrenia*, he presents the case for using large doses of vitamin B-3 to treat acute and chronic schizophrenia. In his book *What Really Causes Schizophrenia*, Professor Foster describes the current state of our knowledge about this widespread condition. What follows is an overview of clinical data detailed in these publications.

Blind, Controlled Studies

As Director of Psychiatric Research in Saskatchewan for the Department of Public Health, Dr Hoffer supervised six blind therapeutic trials with schizophrenic patients during the period 1952 to 1960. This was the first time that blind, controlled trials were used in psychiatric research history, a design adopted on the advice of Dr Bud Fisher, a member of the Canadian Department of Health. The first two trials studied the benefits of a yeast nucleotide preparation in the treatment of schizophrenia. Results were negative. The remaining six focused on vitamin B-3, both niacin and niacinamide. These trials were followed by one double-blind confirmatory report by J.R. Wittenborn[3] and many other reports in the clinical literature.[4]

NAD given in 1-gram doses (though not NADH, which was not available at the time) was usually and very quickly effective in the treatment of schizophrenia when prepared so that it would not be destroyed by stomach acid.

The statistics were conclusive: 90% of schizophrenic patients who had been sick less than 2 years recovered when treated for 2 years by orthomolecular means, including high doses of vitamin B-3. The same recovery rate applied to patients who had responded to standard treatment but had relapsed. Recovery, in this case, means that patients are free of symptoms and signs, that they are getting on well with their family and the community, and that they are paying income tax or are productive members of society in other ways.

In comparison, about 50% of schizophrenic patients who are given the three basics of proper treatment for any disease – adequate housing, good nutrition, and compassion, respect, and dignity – will recover. In contrast, adult schizophrenics who are treated with drugs alone and who do not receive these three basic necessities have a recovery rate below 10%.

To illustrate, in October 27, 2000, King County in Washington State passed a very unusual ordinance,[5] directing psychiatrists to make their patients well and to report annually on how successful those working in the state mental health system had been in achieving this goal. King County spent more than $900 million on mental health the following year in 2001. According to the first mandated report,[6] this was spent on treating 7,831 mental patients, mainly schizophrenics and patients with major depression during the year. Of these 6,949 (88.7%) showed no change, 597 displayed some improvement, 285 (4%) regressed, and four (0.05%) recovered. Put another way, if you suffered from schizophrenia, major depression, or other mental illness in King County during 2001, your chance of a full recovery was less than one in one thousand. The residents of the Seattle area are paying over $22 million for each mental health recovery.

Case Studies

The evidence gathered during the subsequent 50 years concerning the efficacy of vitamin B-3 as a treatment for schizophrenia is very large. In the early 1970s, at one of the last meetings of the Committee on Therapy of the American Schizophrenia Association, the main pioneers of the use of vitamin B-3 concluded that collectively they had successfully treated about 60,000 schizophrenia patients. These included both early and late cases, some of whom had been followed for many years.[7] Not only has vitamin B-3 been shown to be effective for 'acute' schizophrenia (two years after onset), but also for chronic schizophrenia, although the results are not as immediate or dramatic.

Since 1952, Dr Hoffer has treated over 5,000 schizophrenic patients, including many suffering from chronic schizophrenia. Auslander and

Jeste[8] found that only 8% of a population of 155 chronic middle-aged and elderly schizophrenic outpatients living independently were well. The recovery of chronic patients depends on the duration of their illness, the kind of treatments received, and the quality of their care. Dr Hoffer has treated a few patients who had been sick over half their life spans before orthomolecular treatment began and who needed a further 20 years or longer to regain a state of good health. Unfortunately, having lost their most productive years to the illness, they were unable to re-establish themselves as fully productive members of society. Recovery is possible for some chronic schizophrenics, but the road to recovery is not smooth.

Take the case of J.S., a young man who journeyed through the fog, confusion and debilitation of chronic schizophrenia before being treated for 7 years with orthomolecular medicine, including large doses of vitamin B-3. Prior to this young man's first schizophrenic episode and subsequent hospitalization at age 18, there had been no obvious warning signs detected by his parents, except that there was a history of mental illness in his family, validating the hereditary aspect of this disease. His grandmother on his father's side was diagnosed with manic depression, while his aunt on his mother's side was institutionalized with schizophrenia and she died at an early age. Beyond this, neither the medical community nor the educational system had recognized any of his subtle, early pre-episode signals.

During his senior year of high school, his ability to concentrate, express thoughts, and execute what for many would be considered simple tasks were becoming extremely limited. He gave up his part-time job so that he could focus more on his school work and athletic endeavors. That meant that he could no longer afford to drive his car, lacking money for gasoline and car insurance. This logic was received positively by his parents, who thought it represented responsible thinking. He then ceased all activities, except school work. Eventually, this, too, exceeded his capabilities. He was abruptly stricken with schizophrenia and hospitalized for 11 days.

J.S. experienced the traditional cycle of comprehensive testing, with heavy medications and tranquilizers prescribed during this episode. His parents were told that they would need to be prepared for their son to be in and out of hospitals for the rest of his life. They were counseled that the debilitating aspects of the disease could spill over and destroy the family.

Upon his first release from the hospital, J.S. was on three different medications with multiple side-effects and slept up to 20 hours daily. His parents felt that this treatment regimen was taking their son and their family down a road they no longer wanted to travel. As the result of diligent and persistent research by his mother, they identified orthomolecular medicine as a promising alternative, despite the fact that the traditional medical community was highly skeptical. Seven long years later at the age of 25, after following an orthomolecular treatment plan, J.S. began the exciting re-entry process into society and is now a promising young graphic artist.

While still receiving orthomolecular treatment, J.S. is using only one primary medication, at a dosage that is well below the traditionally recommended maintenance level. As a consequence, he is free from the devastating side effects from higher levels. The components of this young man's orthomolecular therapy are consistent with Dr Abram Hoffer's well-known nutritional and megadose vitamin therapy, with its emphasis on vitamin B-3 combined with EPA, as advocated by D. Horrobin,[9] R. Emsley,[10] M. Peet,[11] and their colleagues.

At reduced dosage, traditional medication has been effective in silencing the debilitating aspects of the disease's 'hot/positive' symptoms – that is, his delusions and hallucinations – while the orthomolecular therapies, including the EPA, have neutralized his 'cold/negative' symptoms – that is, his ability to process thoughts along with verbalizing them, the lack of desire to socialize and interact with others, and the drive to accomplish a set goal or objective.

At one point during his 7-year treatment, the megadose vitamin therapy, with its emphasis on vitamin B-3, was suspended for a short period in favor of an alternative. Within 1 week of stopping his vitamin therapy, the cold/negative symptoms of the disease began to re-appear. Vitamin therapy was immediately resumed, and within days the symptoms of the disease again were under control.

For some who suffer chronically from this disease, orthomolecular medicine and nutritional therapies alone can take the place of the strong medications utilized by the traditional medical community. Identifying the presence of various food allergies, heavy metals, and nutritional deficiencies, combined with targeted nutritional therapies, also allow many chronic schizophrenics to recover.

At a *Food as Medicine* conference in 2003, just before Dr Hoffer was about to speak, a physician from the audience came to the front of the room, turned to the audience, and began to cry. After she had calmed down, she apologized to the group and said that, whenever she told her story, she could not stop crying. These were tears of happiness, not sadness.

Thirty years ago her older brother was schizophrenic and not responding well to conventional treatment. Their father called Dr Hoffer to learn about orthomolecular treatment. Soon after his son was treated with nutrients, he recovered, became a lawyer, raised a family, and has been well since. His sister was crying because of the terror that afflicted her family when her brother was not responding to conventional treatment and to the joy they felt because he had become normal.

Dr Hoffer has collected a series of 18 similar accounts written by recovered patients who became highly productive members of our society. All were treatment failures on drugs alone.[12] On an orthomolecular program, with large doses of vitamin B-3, six of these patients are now university students, one practices medicine, and others include a professional artist, an engineer, a teacher, a poet, and a writer. Five are business professionals. In late August 2004, Dr Hoffer received a letter from a patient who started treatment with an orthomolecular protocol in early 2001; at that time he was 21 years old. "I have just been accepted to a medical school," he wrote, "and have almost completely recovered."

The human costs of schizophrenia to patients and their families is impossible to calculate. How do you estimate this loss? The significance of this cost can only be understood by patients and their families who have been freed from the ravages of this disease. The rest of us can only imagine their costs by reading the accounts of patients who have recovered.

Social Consequences

Clearly, inadequate conventional treatment of schizophrenics costs society many gifted people, not simply their potential talent but also their very lives. With the exception of those undergoing orthomolecular treatment, schizophrenic patients kill themselves at an unusually high rate. However, not one of the 5,000 schizophrenic patients under Dr Hoffer's care has committed suicide. When one young patient relapsed and was admitted to hospital, his treating psychiatrist refused to continue the vitamin program and prescribed only drugs. A few months after discharge, this patient killed himself.

Not only does vitamin B-3 treatment reduce the incidence of suicide, orthomolecular therapy markedly decreases the number of re-admissions to hospital. The cost savings to the healthcare system are enormous. Modern psychiatry argues that once schizophrenics have been stabilized on antipsychotic drugs, they must continue them for life because of risk of relapse. This is a new principle in medicine. One does not keep a patient who has been treated with penicillin for pneumonia on the antibiotic forever, just to prevent a relapse sometime in the future. For schizophrenic patients, it is better to have been well for a long time with a slight risk of relapse than be subjected to continuous drug toxicity.

Olanzapine, for example, increases the risk of developing diabetes mellitus and, as a result, schizophrenic patients using it become diabetic. Which is the more acceptable risk to patients, preventing them from becoming normal and allowing them to become diabetic, or taking then off olanzapine when they are well without it and increasing their risk of relapsing, especially when they can be easily treated for schizophrenia again?

In Canada, enforced medication is now enshrined in law. The current legislation ensures that schizophrenics are kept heavily tranquilized, sick, and unproductive under drug control, denying them the freedoms guaranteed by the Charter of Rights. During a conditional discharge or extended leave from hospital, patients are forced to remain on drugs. If they refuse to take them, they are forcibly returned to hospital. Given antipsychotic drugs, fewer than 10% of schizophrenics ever become gainfully employed.

As reported in a study of 42 medical doctors who became schizophrenic and were given nothing but drugs, only 12 went back to practice. This was possible for six of them because they were married to nurses who helped maintain the practice. Dr Hoffer has treated three physicians who were schizophrenic. They all recovered and changed the focus of their practices to become orthomolecular doctors.

Lack of adequate treatment also fails to prevent the criminal behavior of a few patients whose illness is not managed in time. Many years ago a study in England of 200 convicted murderers demonstrated that the majority were schizophrenic. About 35 years ago, Dr Hoffer examined 12 of the most difficult prisoners in Prince Albert Penitentiary in Saskatchewan and found that nine of them were paranoid schizophrenics. This does not mean that patients with schizophrenia are any more prone to criminal and antisocial behavior than the general population. However, when schizophrenic patients do commit a crime, it often has that 'particularly difficult to understand' quality seen in multiple murders or random shootings. Children who 'shoot up' their schools and citizens who shoot their presidents tend to be schizophrenic because these bizarre acts are usually the product of a disorganized brain.

Society is already well aware of the relationships between uncontrolled schizophrenia and bizarre incomprehensible anti-social behavior. In today's paper, for example, there is a report of two retired physicians (husband and wife) who have been found murdered. The police are looking for their son, who lived nearby and is schizophrenic. If schizophrenics are treated effectively they will not commit such terrible crimes. Unfortunately, society equates all incomprehensible and bizarre crimes with schizophrenia. This is a major disservice to the 99% of such patients who are as law abiding as the general public.

Schizophrenics should not be ostracized for the fact that a very small percentage of them commit such acts, any more than society in general can be blamed for those members who commit criminal anti-social activities. Indeed, if all schizophrenic patients were diagnosed early and treated with orthomolecular medicine, the majority of such terrible acts could be avoided.

Take the case of a young university student who was referred to Dr Hoffer for assessment and therapy. N.W. took his rifle, drove to the outskirts of the city, and began to shoot at cars traveling along the road. Fortunately, no one was hurt. He was arrested and charged. His lawyer sensed there was something abnormal about him, and he was referred to Dr Hoffer. This student was working on his doctorate. He recalled a series of previous anti-social acts. On one occasion, for example, he stayed in the Library of Congress in Washington, DC, until its doors were locked and then pushed over numerous book stacks. He described this activity without emotion.

N.W.'s lawyer was advised that he was schizophrenic and that he needed to be treated. Dr Hoffer began to see him every 2 weeks. After the third month, he came to the interview very agitated, anxious, in a cold sweat. He had suddenly realized that by shooting at cars he might have killed someone. He had regained insight. In response, the courts were compassionate.

The charges were stayed and he was allowed to complete his degree. He became a university professor.

From these cases and many others in Dr Hoffer's and his colleagues' case files, orthomolecular treatment is clearly effective for even chronic schizophrenia. Many patients recover fully, others are much improved, few are not positively affected. None are worse.

Some chronic patients will require small does of medication to complement the nutrient therapy, others will not. This does not mean that patients will be able to escape from seeing psychiatrists at regular intervals. If they are on medication, it is mandatory that they be followed to ensure they come to no harm from the drugs. In addition, problems arise now and then, as they do with any group of patients who have a chronic disease, for example, diabetes mellitus.

Orthomolecular treatment is safe, even when used for many years. No major side effects are caused by the small doses of tranquilizers that many of these patients still require. The program does not produce tranquilizer psychosis.

Schizophrenic patients find the program palatable and most remain compliant. They are able to look forward to continuing improvement.

References

[1] Public Health Agency of Canada. A Report on Mental Illnesses in Canada. Chap 3: Schizophrenia.

[2] Answers.com . Schizophrenia. http//www.Answers.com/Topic/Schizophrenia

[3] Pfeiffer, C.C. Mental and Elemental Nutrients. New Canaan, CT: Keats Publishing Inc., 1975.

[4] Foster HD. What Really Causes Shizophrenia. Victoria, BC: Trafford Publishing, 2003.

[5] Hoffer A. Vitamin B-3 and Schizophrenia. Discovery, Recovery Controversy. Kingston, ON: Quarry Health Books, 1998.

[6] Hoffer A, Osmond H: How To Live With Schizophrenia. New York, NY: University Books, 1966; new and revised edition, New York, NY Citadel Press:

1992; revised by Hoffer A as Healing Schizophrenia. Toronto, ON: CCNM Press, 2004.

7 Foster HD. What Really Causes Shizophrenia. Victoria, BC: Trafford Publishing, 2003.

8 Wittenborn JR. A Search for responders to niacin supplementation. Archives Gen Psychiatry 1974;31:547-552

9 Hoffer A. Treatment Manual. Toronto, ON: International Schizophrenia Foundation, 2007.

10 Safe Harbor. Alternative Mental Health On-line. King County, WA. Ordinance Requiring Psychiatrists to Make People Well. Passed October 16,2000. Ordinance 13974. Sponsors: Pullen, Fimia,Grossett, and Irons. http://www.alternativementalhealth.com/articles/article.KingCounty.htm

11 Safe Harbor. Alternative Mental Health News, Issue 28, November 2002. County Mental Health System Achieves Almost No Recoveries. ezine@alternativemenalhealth.com

12 Hawkins DR. The prevention of tardive dyskinesia with high dosage vitamins of 58,000 patients. Journal Orthomolecular Medicine 1986;1:24-26.

13 Auslander LA and Jeste DV. Sustained remission of schizophrenia among community-dwelling older patients. Am Journal Psychiarry 2004;161:1490-93.

14 Horrobin D, Jenkins K, Bennett S, and Vankar GK. Eicosapentaenoic acid and arachidonic acid. Collaboration and not antagonism is the key to biologic understanding. Prostaglandins. Leukot Essential Fatty Acids 2002;66:83-90.

15 Emsley R, Myburgh C, Oosthuizen P, and van Rensburg SJ. Randomized, placebo- controlled study of ethyl-eicosapentaenoic acid as a supplement treatment in schizophrenia. Am J Psychiatry 2002;159(9):1596-98.

16 Peet M, Brind J, Ramchand CN,and Vankar GK. Two double-blind placebo-controlled studies of eicosapentaenoic acid in the treatment of schizophrenia. Schizophrenia Research 2001;49(3):243-51.

17 The Center for Mind-Body Medicine in Association with The University of Minnesota and Georgetown University School of Medicine. Food as Medicine:

Integrating Nutrition into Clinical Practice and Medical Education. Sponsored by The Wallace Research Foundation and the Hilton Family Foundation. Marriott Bay Point Resort, Panama City Beach, Florida. March 2-8, 2003.

[18] Hoffer A: Mental Health Regained. Toronto, ON: International Schizophrenia Foundation, 2007.

PYROLURIA

Prevalence

Pyroluria appears to be a medical condition that is indicative, not of a specific illness, but rather of high levels of oxidative stress.[1] Pyroluria is identified by an excess of pyrroles in human urine and occurs most frequently in schizophrenics, although it is commonly seen in other illnesses, including ADHD, autism, alcoholism, and depression.[2]

In 1965, O'Reilly and Hughes claimed that pyroluria was present in 11% of healthy controls, 24% of disturbed children, 42% of psychiatric patients, and 52% of schizophrenics.[3] Dr Hoffer's experience after testing a much larger sample consisting of "thousands of patients at our four research centers" was somewhat different.[4] Elevated "kryptopyrrole" was found in the urine of 75% of acute schizophrenics, 25% of all non-psychotic patients, and 5% of physically ill patients. It was absent from the urine of normal subjects, and, most interestingly, was never found in the urine of recovered schizophrenics.

The evidence suggests that although urinary kryptopyrrole (probably 2-hydroxy-hemopyrrolene-5-one) is not an absolute sign of schizophrenia, it occurs with much greater regularity in schizophrenics than in anyone else.

Role of Vitamin B-3

In 1960, the Saskatchewan research team directed by Dr Hoffer was ana-lyzing urine from schizophrenic patients, hoping to find something unique that might be used to characterize this condition. They were using a newly developed technique called paper chromatography, but with lim-ited success. Dr Hoffer hypothesized that perhaps LSD might produce a chemical in the body that would be such a marker. The psychotomimetic experience caused by this hallucinogen seemed similar to that of the schiz-ophrenic syndrome. LSD might, therefore, induce the body to produce some chemical that was similar to one that might be naturally present in the bodies of schizophrenics.

At the time, Dr Hoffer was routinely treating alcoholics with LSD, using the psychedelic experience as a form of treatment. To test the possibility that LSD might cause the body to produce a chemical similar to that cre-ated in schizophrenia, one alcoholic patient was given 200 mcg of LSD. A urine sample was taken before and then again 2 hours later at the height of the LSD experience. These samples were examined using paper chro-matography.

The next day, the chemically treated paper strip used to measure the urine sample taken during the LSD experience displayed a mauve spot at RF 0.80. This mauve spot did not appear on the paper strip measuring the initial sample. After the laboratory had shown that the substance on the paper was not LSD itself or a derivative of it, urine from schizophrenic patients was tested in a similar manner. It was discovered that this mauve substance was much more commonly found in the urine of schizophren-ics than in normal controls, but it also occurred in a smaller proportion of children with learning disorders and in patients with depression and anx-iety. It was present also on some cases of cancer, especially that of the lung. This mauve spot could also be detected in samples from the siblings of a few schizophrenics. Clearly, this was not a diagnostic test for schizophre-nia, but it did establish the presence of an unusual substance in the urine of many of the mentally ill.

When clinical comparisons are made, 'mauve factor' patients are found to resemble schizophrenics more than they do patients with depression or anxiety states. More importantly, they respond very well to large doses of vitamin B-3, as do schizophrenic patients. Subsequent research showed that supplemental pyridoxine and zinc were also very important in the treatment of all mauve-positive patients.

Clinical Evidence

These successes led to studies of this phenomenon in thousands of patients in four Saskatchewan hospitals. The results were reported in detail in the *Journal of Neuropsychiatry* in 1961.[5]

Later, in association with Dr Carl C. Pfeiffer, working with Dr Humphry Osmond in New Jersey, the chemical nature of the substance was identified. Dr Pfeiffer discovered it to be tightly bound zinc and pyridoxine that produced a double deficiency of both nutrients.[6] Pfeiffer clinically described as kryptopyrroleuria the condition Osmond and Hoffer had previously called malvaria. Subsequently, his quantitative test has been enormously valuable in laboratories, where its presence is used to diagnose and to assist in developing treatment. Beyond this, Hoffer observed that cancer patients who tested positive for kryptopyrrole urea and who excreted large amounts of zinc and pyridoxine had a better prognosis and lived longer when treated by standard methods than those who did not.[7]

And there the matter rested. The psychiatric research professions did not follow up with any examination of claims about the significance of kryptopyrrole. They also confused the mauve factor with another substance that erroneously had been claimed to be present in schizophrenic urine. Nevertheless, Dr Hoffer continued to use this test for many years, as did Dr H. Riordan and Dr William Walsh at the Brain Bio Center in Chicago.

Luckily the story does not end there. The concept has been slowly gaining intellectual support, with Dr Woody McGinnis now coordinating studies of the mauve factor.[8,9] The chemical structure originally postulated has been found to be incorrect, but it is close enough to reality to be useful clinically. The chemical, often excreted in the urine of the mentally ill, is hydroxyhemoppyrrolin-2-one, a member of the pyrrole group. It is still often referred to as the mauve factor, the original term. It is found not only in urine, but also in blood and cerebrospinal fluid. It is not stable in light and heat, and must be stabilized with ascorbic acid unless it is measured immediately.

The presence of the mauve factor is a useful predictor of higher needs for pyridoxine and zinc. Many clinicians in Europe now use the Mauve assay to manage somatic health problems. McGinnis suggests that it is a biomarker for oxidative stress. This being the case, it is not surprising that anti-oxidants are therapeutic. Some of the anti-oxidants include zinc, pyridoxine and the NAD-NADH system.

The NAD-NADH system, so important in the prevention of pellagra, is a very active oxidation reduction mechanism. It may eventually be found to play a significant role in the treatment of diseases characterized by oxidative stress, as may other anti-oxidants, such as vitamin C and E. With so many laboratories now showing interest, further insights are bound to follow.

It is already becoming clearer why cancer patients testing positive for the mauve factor live longer than normal. Cancer tissue tends to become anoxemic and sensitive to oxygen. As a result, chemotherapeutic drugs are strong oxidants. Schizophrenic patients suffer from oxidative stress, thus increasing the production of adrenochrome and similar indoles. These are mitotic poisons and, in schizophrenia, seem to cause a decreased incidence of cancer.[10] It is generally agreed that schizophrenic patients, as well as other patients with many chronic diseases, are under increased oxidative stress. This is made worse if natural anti-oxidants, such as glutathione, are deficient. This is true for schizophrenia because glutathione neutralizes adrenochrome.

Is it possible that cancer patients who test positive for the mauve factor were controlling their cancer more effectively due to increased levels of oxidative stress and higher concentrations of adrenochrome. In the presence of anti-oxidants, this oxidative stress would be more toxic to tumors than to normal tissues. It would be interesting to study a large sample of cancer patients for mauve factors to see if its presence does increase life expectancy.

References

[1] Heleniak E, Lamola S. A new prostaglandin disturbance syndrome in schizophrenia: delta-6-pyroluria. Medical Hypotheses 1986;19(4):333-38.

[2] Hoffer A. Adventures in Psychiatry. The Scientific Memoirs or Dr. Abram Hoffer. Caledon, ON: KOS Publishing Inc., 2005.

3 O'Reilly and Hughes, cited by Pfeiffer CC, Mailloux R, Forsythe L. The Schizo-phrenias: Ours to Conquer. Wichita, KS: Bio-Communications Press, 1988.

4 Hoffer A. Vitamin B3 and Schizophrenia: Discovery, Recovery, Controversy. Kingston, ON: Quarry Press, 1998.

5 Hoffer A and Mahon M. The presence of unidentified substances in the urine of psychiatric patients. J of Neuropsychiatry 1961;2:287-374.

6 Pfeiffer, C.C. Mental and Elemental Nutrients. New Canaan, CT: Keats Publishing Inc., 1975.

7 Hoffer A, Pauling L. Healing Cancer: Complementary Vitamin & Drug Treatments. Toronto, ON: CCNM Press, 2004.

8 McGinnis WR. Urinary pyrrole (Mauve Factor): Metric for oxidative stress in behavioral disorders. Linus Pauling Institute 2nd International Conference on Diet and Optimum Health. Abstract 34. Portland, Oregon. May 21-4, 2003.

9 McGinnis WR. Urinary pyrrole ('Mauve Factor'): Marker for oxidative stress. Presentation and syllabus narrative for the American College for Advancement of Medicine Spring Conference. Orlando, Florida. May 20-22, 2004.

10 Foster HD, Hoffer A. Schizophrenia and cancer: The adrenochrome balanced morphism. Medical Hypotheses 2004;62,415-419.

ADDICTIONS

Prevalence

In the United States, there are an estimated 15.1 million alcoholics, 4.6 million of whom are women.[1] In addition, 19.5 million Americans over the age of 12 use illegal drugs and 19,000 die from this habit each year. Beyond this, according to the Centers for Disease Control and Prevention, 44.5 million U.S. adults were current smokers in 2004, more than 1 out of 5 Americans.[2] In any given year, almost half of these smokers attempt to give up the habit, in most cases unsuccessfully.

According to the Canadian Centre on Substance Abuse, Canada incurs $40 billion in annual costs as a consequence of drug addiction.[3] Tobacco, for example, costs Canadian taxpayers an estimated $17 billion annually, while alcohol-related expenditures are $14.6 billion and illicit-drug costs $8.2 billion. In total, 43,162 Canadians died from addiction-associated causes in 2002, with tobacco use being responsible for 37,209 of those deaths.

Alcoholism

Role of Vitamin B-3

In the 1950s, Dr Hoffer and his colleagues in Saskatchewan began to treat large numbers of schizophrenic patients with high doses of vitamin B-3. A few of these patients were both alcoholic and schizophrenic. From this group, it was learned that, coincidentally, niacin was a particularly good treatment for alcohol addiction.[4]

This is not too surprising because many alcoholics have an abnormal allele that results in the production of an ineffective form of aldehyde dehydrogenase. As a result, they are genetically incapable of the normal oxidation of acetaldehyde, which builds up in their blood. This increases their susceptibility to alcoholism, but can be mitigated by high doses of niacin. Alcoholism is a NAD deficiency disease, and niacin can reduce the alcoholic's addiction.

Dr Roger Williams has called alcoholism a genetotrophic disease, with "geneto" referring to genetics or hereditary factors, while trophic implies dietary and nutritional factors.[5,6] Williams pointed out that most alcoholics are deficient in nutrients because alcoholic drinks, at best, contain very low levels. Eight ounces a day of whiskey dilutes the diet by about 20%. As a result, an alcoholic would have to increase the intake of nutrients by 20% to make up for this loss. However, they very rarely consume nutritious foods. This is one of the reasons that alcoholics respond so well to niacin and other nutrients – they are suffering from numerous self-induced nutritional deficiencies.

Clinical Evidence

In one case, a patient had joined Alcoholics Anonymous (AA) in order to stop drinking, but, whenever she succeeded, she would begin to hear voices, a symptom which was worse than the consequences of drinking. She would then begin to drink again to get rid of these voices. Clearly, she was confronted with a terrible dilemma. Should she be a sober member of AA and suffer auditory hallucinations, or should she be free of hallucinations and be an out-of-control alcoholic? Dr Hoffer offered her a third choice, starting her on high-dose niacin therapy. Within a few months, she was able to stay sober without any recurrence of hallucinations. Later, she became a member of the first Schizophrenics Anonymous group Dr Hoffer had helped organize in Saskatoon in 1960, with the support and advice of Bill W., the cofounder of Alcoholics Anonymous.

Around this time, Hoffer realized that alcoholics did not have to be schizophrenic in order to respond positively to elevated niacin. He shared this insight in the early 1960s with Bill W., who started taking 1 g of niacin, three times daily. As a result, he was relieved of severe exhaustion, tension, anxiety, and insomnia in 2 weeks.

Soon after, Bill W. persuaded 30 friends who attended Alcoholics Anonymous in New York to take niacin. One third of them were relieved of their depression after 1 month, another third after 2 months, but the remaining third were not affected. However, Bill W.'s enthusiasm for niacin treatment got him into 'hot water' at international AA headquarters. To inform doctors treating alcoholics and fellow AA members of the value of niacin, he was forced to go outside the established medical system. The Huxley Institute of Biosocial Research, founded by Humphry Osmond and with Abram Hoffer at the time as its president, gave Bill W. a small grant to cover his out-of-pocket expenses while he prepared several newsletters for AA doctors.[7] These doctors quickly became very enthusiastic, and niacin started to be used on an increasing scale to help alcoholics regain their physical and mental health.

Dr R.F. Smith, the medical director of a hospital in Detroit that specialized in the treatment of alcoholics, began to promote niacin for treating alcoholism.[8,9]. The response rate of patients treated with vitamin B-3 was very high, as shown in the following summary of his results.

The patients initially treated with niacin wanted to stop drinking, but there were also other alcoholics in the study who had no desire to give up the habit. Nevertheless, they agreed that they would take the niacin anyway. After a few years, more and more of this group were drinking less. This is not surprising. Relaxed and healthy individuals will very rarely become alcoholic. They must first have a problem that allows alcohol to make them feel better.

Niacin has many other benefits for alcoholics. It can, for example, protect the liver against the excess of alcohol. Rat studies have demonstrated that a single dose of alcohol, equivalent to one that would make an adult

	Year	Number of Alcoholics Treated with Vitamin B-3	Percent with Good and Excellent Response
Outpatients	1967	239	63
	1968	233	81
	1969	214	91
	1970	194	100
Hospital Patients	1967	216	73
	1968	191	75
	1969	174	89
	1970	164	100
Sanitarium Patients	1967	52	69
	1968	50	84
	1969	49	94
	1970	48	94

man legally drunk, caused an accumulation of fat in animal livers within 8 hours.[10,11] When the rats were first given elevated niacin (equivalent to 17 g of niacin for a 150-lb human), there was no such liver fat deposition.

Niacin is clearly one of the nutrients that alcoholics need, but there are others, likely including the remaining B vitamins and omega-3 essential fatty acid. Indeed, it is highly likely that alcoholics are deficient in almost all essential nutrients. As with the other syndromes described in this book, niacin should not be prescribed alone. Attention must also be paid to diet to eliminate as much as possible the intake of free sugars and to check for food allergies. Vitamin C and some of the other B vitamins need to be taken as supplements, if necessary, as well as the omega-3 essential fatty acids. In orthomolecular medicine, there are no one-nutrient, one-disease treatments.

Clinical experience during the past 40 years has shown that niacin works best when it is given to members of Alcoholics Anonymous or patients otherwise motivated to stop drinking. To gain the full benefit of this vitamin, patients must be sober. For most of them, it removes the severe tension, agitation, and insomnia many still suffer even though they are abstinent.

Fetal Alcohol Syndrome

T he sins of parents are often visited upon their children. This applies particularly to fetal alcohol syndrome, where a metabolic derangement in
the fetus is caused by a mother's use of alcohol during pregnancy. This can
result in many physical and psychological disorders in the child. While
prevention by abstaining from alcohol during pregnancy is an obvious
solution to this problem, there appears to be no simple effective treatment.

However, Dr Hoffer has treated several of these children with success
using a multivitamin program. A key in this treatment protocol is vitamin
B-3. LR, born in May 1994 and seen September 2004, had been diagnosed
with fetal alcohol syndrome. Her great aunt took her for care. She had
been neglected by her birth mother, later counseled, but she continued to
have major difficulty in focusing. She would have to be asked the same
question over and over again. She learned slowly and suffered mood
swings. She was hyper-vigilant and physically aggressive toward her
younger sister. Dexedrine made her much worse, causing severe night-
mares and visual illusions, and Ritalin, which is less toxic than Dexedrine,
did not have any therapeutic effect.

Her aunt had placed her on a dairy-free diet program, which produced a
major improvement. Dr Hoffer added niacin (100 mg after each meal),
ascorbic acid (500 mg after each meal), the essential fatty acids, and a multivitamin complex. She did not like the niacin flush, so her B-3 was changed
to inositol niacinate (no flush niacin) 500 mg, three times daily. When seen
10 months later, she was almost normal. Because she had lost so much valuable learning experience, her aunt planned to have her go to a special school
where she would be able to receive more attention from her teachers. She
was cheerful, relaxed, and well on the way to complete recovery.

Interestingly, Ieraci and Herrera have recently shown that nicotinamide
can help protect against ethanol-induced neurodegeneration in the developing mouse brain if given soon after exposure to alcohol.[12]

Drug Addictions

D rug addicts also are treatable with large doses of niacin. About 40 years
ago, while on a speaking tour of California, Dr Hoffer addressed a

meeting in a church hall in Los Angeles. After this talk, several Chicano leaders came forward and told him they were routinely giving some of their heroin-addicted friends very large doses of niacin, who responded very well to it with greatly reduced withdrawal symptoms. This information was interesting, but not conclusive. Similar reports also appeared in medical literature, authored by Dr Irwin Stone and Dr A.F. Libby.[13] Although the data was much more persuasive, this approach to drug addiction has not been pursued.

At this point, the niacin-drug addiction story takes a strange turn. Many years ago, Dr Hoffer received a copy of a note sent by L. Ron Hubbard, the founder of the Church of Scientology, to some of his supporters. Mr Hubbard advised his followers to take niacin, but did not indicate why. Later, Dr Hoffer became aware of what scientologists were calling the Hubbard detoxification technique. This involved using wet or dry heat in saunas to cause heavy sweating. Before entering the sauna, scientologists were taking niacin so that the associated flush and sweating coincided. Niacin would drive the body's toxins into the perspiration so that they could be rinsed away.

Although this is an interesting hypothesis, it has not been examined seriously by the medical profession, chiefly because of a skeptical attitude toward scientology, not because of its therapeutic merits. In 1998, under the title "Scientology Unmasked," Joseph Mallia argued that the promotion of this detoxification program using niacin was merely an attempt to enhance and expand the influence of the Church of Scientology. Nevertheless, during the past few years, the Second Chance Program for prison inmates has used the Hubbard technique to help a large number of prison inmates recover from their drug addictions.[14] These results, if they can be corroborated, are very impressive.

Saunas have been used for centuries, and many users claim that they improve health. Similarly, many people who suffer from subclinical pellagra also feel better when taking niacin. The basic research question to be answered is whether sauna use and niacin supplementation taken together are more beneficial to health than either of the two treatments taken independently.

LSD

Within a few years of the onset of the psychedelic movement in North America, the most commonly used hallucinogen was LSD. In 1952, only about five substances were known to be hallucinogens and none were widely available. Today, the number of such drugs in use has increased enormously. If LSD, 'magic mushrooms', mescaline, and amphetamine-type substances are taken, this can lead to a schizophrenic syndrome.

Niacin is a very good antidote against LSD. Niacin reverses both the effect of adrenochrome as seen on the electroencephalogram in human subjects and the psychotomimetic effect of adrenochrome given intravenously. We know of no reports of the use of niacin for other hallucinogens.

During the period when Dr Hoffer and his colleagues were treating alcoholic patients with the psychedelic experience, they used 100 mg of intravenous niacin if the LSD reaction was slow to subside. Niacin is better than tranquilizers since it does not leave the patients groggy and disoriented. If the patients were not fully out of the experience, they were given 500 mg of niacin to take as needed. In every case, they were warned about the expected flush so that they would not become anxious about it. These study results are included in the 1967 landmark book publication, *The Hallucinogens*, by Dr Abram Hoffer and his colleague, Dr Humphry Osmond.[15]

Nicotine Addiction

Chemically, nicotine and niacin are quite similar. Indeed, the vitamin niacin can be made from nicotine by splitting open the second side ring. It is not surprising, therefore, that niacin has been used to treat this form of addiction. Dr J.E. Prousky gave seven patients daily doses of niacin, ranging from 1.5 to 3 g.[16] Two of these patients stopped smoking cigarettes within 2 to 3 weeks. The other five halved their tobacco intake. Nicotine probably attaches to the same brain receptors as niacin. If this is correct, flooding the brain with niacin should mitigate the effects of nicotine. Obviously, this is a possible treatment for nicotine addiction that requires much more attention.

References

1 Wrong Diagnosis? Prevalence and Incidence of Drug Abuse. http://www.wrongdiagnosis.com/d/drug°abuse/prevalence.htm

2 American Cancer Society. Cigarette Smoking. http://www.cancer.org/docroot/ PED/content/PED°10°2X°Cigarette°Smoking.asp

3 Canadian Centre on Substance Abuse. The Costs of Substance Abuse in Canada 2002. http://www.ccsa.ca/CCSA/EN/Research/Research°Activities/TheCost

4 Hoffer A. Adventures in Psychiatry. The Scientific Memoirs of Dr. Abram Hoffer. Caledon, Ontario: KOS Publishing Inc. 2005.

5 Williams RJ. Nutrition and Alcoholism. Norman, Oklahoma: University of Oklahoma Press, 1951.

6 Williams RJ. Alcoholism: The Nutritional Approach. Austin, Texas: University of Texas Press, 1959.

7 Smith RF. Niacin and the Alcoholic. In: The Vitamin B-3 Therapy. A Third Communication to A.A. Physicians. Edited by Bill W. January 1971.

8 Smith RF. A five-year trial of massive nicotinic acid therapy of alcoholics in Michigan. Journal of Orthomolecular Psychiatry 1974;3:327-31.

9 Smith RF. Alcoholism and criminal behavior. In: Hippchen LJ (ed.). Holistic Approaches to Offender Rehabilitation. Springfield, IL: CC Thomas, 1982.

10 French SW, Miyamoto K, Tsukamoto H. Ethanol-induced hepatic fibrosis in the rat. Role of the amount of dietary fat. Alcoholism: Clinical and Experimental Research 1985;10(6):13s-19s.

11 National Institute on Alcohol Abuse and Alcoholism of the National Institute of Health. Animal Models in Alcohol Research. NIAAA Alcohol Alert, No 24 PH 350. April 1994.

12 Ieraci A, Herrera DG. Nicotinamide protects against ethanol-induced apoptotic neurodegeneration in the developing mouse brain. PLOS Med. 2006;3(4):e101.

[13] Libby AF, Stone I. The hypoascorbemia-Kwashiorkor approach to drug addiction therapy: A pilot study. Journal of Orthomolecular Psychiatry 1977;6:300-08.

[14] The Second Chance Program. Prison-based rehabilitation. La Mesa, CA. http://www.penalrehab.org/

[15] Hoffer A, Osmond H. The Hallucinogens. New York: Academic Press. 1967.

[16] Prousky JE. Vitamin B-3 for nicotine addiction. J Orthomolecular Medicine 2004;19:56-57.

CARDIOVASCULAR, CORONARY, AND CEREBROVASCULAR DISEASES

Prevalence

Throughout the developed world, at most ages, diseases of the heart and stroke compete with cancer as the major cause of death. In Canada, for men of all ages, 36% of deaths are attributable to cardiovascular disease, while for women the mortality is even higher, at 39%.[1] In 1995, there were 79,117 deaths attributed to cardiovascular disease, compared to 75,221 in 1992.[2] Coronary heart disease was responsible for the death of 26.4 per 100,000 among American white males in 1992.[3] Each year about 500,000 people in the United States have their first stroke, and about 25% of these die from it. A further 100,000 have a recurrent stroke. There is nothing unique about North America. In England, coronary heart disease kills more than 110,000 people each year. More than 1.4 million suffer from angina, and each year 275,000 people have a heart attack.[4]

Conventional medicine is consistently lowering the acceptable levels of serum cholesterol, but at this time, some 105 million American adults have cholesterol levels above 200 mg/dl. This is considered borderline high. About 37 million of these have values in excess of 240 mg/dl, a level which is definitely considered high.

Role of Vitamin B-3

In 1938, soon after vitamin B-3 was identified as the anti-pellagra factor and its vasodilator properties were observed, Dr L. Condorelli and his associates began to study its therapeutic applications to heart and vascular disease, as well as other related conditions.[5] Condorelli reported the following properties of niacin, given by intravenous injection or by mouth: (1) increase in the velocity of the circulation; (2) increase in cardiac output; (3) increase in systolic stroke volume; (4) decrease in total pulmonary pressure; (5) increase in peripheral circulation in the viscera, brain, and muscles; (6) increase in oxygenation; (7) increase in pulmonary oxygen diffusion; (8) and decrease in EEG abnormalities caused by hypoxia of the myocardium. In short, niacin improves the body's blood flow, improves circulation of oxygen, and restores organ function, without increasing blood pressure. Condorelli also described niacin's therapeutic effect on the following conditions:

- Angiospasms, including headaches and other regional spasms, such as occur in the retina with hypertensive spells (niacin must be given intravenously)
- Spasm in the limbs (except for Raynaud's disease)
- Embolism (relaxed the spastic vessels around the embolus)
- Thrombotic arteriopathies, such as intermittent claudication
- Angina
- Coronary insufficiency
- Eclampsia
- Nephritis

Subsequently, the therapeutic effects of niacin on heart, stroke, and vascular disease have been studied, with significant results. As Dr Robert D. McCracken wrote in a survey of the related literature, "an impressive body of scientific research clearly demonstrates that niacin, when taken in mega quantities, can have a protective and healthful effect upon the cardiovascular system. There can be no doubt about this; the findings are clear and consistent. Enough is known about the biochemical effects of niacin for us to say that niacin exerts a protective effect upon the basic chemistry that researchers believe cause many forms of cardiovascular disease."[6]

Clinical Evidence

Hypercholesterolemia

The discovery that niacin lowered cholesterol levels arose from research conducted by Professor Rudl Altschul, Chair, Department of Anatomy, University of Saskatchewan. Professor Altschul had found that rabbits developed hypercholesterolemia very rapidly if they were fed cooked egg yolk in a specially baked cake. Raw egg yolk did not have the same effect. He also found that exposing rabbits to ultraviolet light decreased their cholesterol levels. Altschul wanted to try ultraviolet light treatment on people, but could not find any doctor in Saskatoon willing to work with him until Dr Hoffer agreed to provide subjects in one of the provincial mental hospitals. Since the treatment was safe and patients could not be harmed by it, he considered that it would be good for these mental patients to mix with healthy young people who would be conducting the research.

At that time, Hoffer himself had been suffering from bleeding gums. Large doses of vitamin C did not help, but after taking niacin for 2 weeks for other reasons, his gums were healed. From this, Hoffer hypothesized that the niacin had increased the rate of repair of gum tissues, which had been under physical stress from maloccluded teeth.

Professor Altschul thought that the most important single pathological factor in coronary disease was the inability of the intima (the inner wall of the blood vessel) to repair itself, especially where the blood stream changed direction, causing the greatest stress to the arteries. As Altschul explained this hypothesis to him, Hoffer recalled his bleeding gums and suggested that niacin might be able to heal the arterial wall's intima. Hoffer then gave the Altschul one pound of crystalline niacin to test the effects on experimental rabbits.

A few months later, Altschul reported back that the niacin had lowered cholesterol levels in these rabbits. On receiving this news, Hoffer organized a study using humans, which revealed similar results in lowering cholesterol levels.[7] Published in 1955, these results were soon corroborated by Dr William Parsons Jr., then at the Mayo Clinic in Rochester, Minnesota.[8] Parsons became a great believer in the value of niacin and wrote the book *Cholesterol Control without Diet! The Niacin Solution*. He considered that niacin was the best substance available to control cholesterol because it decreased the incidence of stroke and coronary disease, thereby extending life expectancy.

There is strong evidence to support these claims. In 1986, the *Journal of the American College of Cardiology* drug coronary study showed that men who experience a coronary and who were then given niacin died less frequently than normal and so lived longer.[9] Specifically, there was a 10% decrease in death rate and a 2-year increase in longevity. Since that time, niacin has become the gold standard for normalizing lipid levels, even though this fact is rarely taught in medical school. Niacin also lowers triglycerides and lipoprotein(a), while elevating HDL (the good cholesterol fraction), which is its most important function. Not only does niacin normalize and stabilize blood lipid levels, it inhibits the release of fatty acids under severe stress.

In a logical world, niacin would be used, at a cost of roughly $10 each month, to lower coronary death rates. However, the statin drugs, roughly ten times as expensive, have the backing of the pharmaceutical companies and continue to play this role. Even when niacin alone is not completely effective, it can be combined with simvastatin.[10,11] This dual treatment approach has produced marked clinical and angiographic benefits for patients with coronary disease and low HDL levels. In contrast, the University of British Columbia Therapeutics Initiative sent a letter to 12,000 British Columbia doctors in 2003 doctors stating that statins "have not been shown to provide an overall health benefit" when prescribed to people who have not already had a stroke or heart attack and do not have cardiovascular disease.[12] More recently, Dr Graveline has reported that statins cause transient global amnesia.[13]

Mitigating Tobacco Use

The use of tobacco is very stressful to the heart. Niacin can mitigate some of its harmful effects, for example, by decreasing the elevation of free fatty acids caused by smoking. In one experiment, free fatty acids rose by 30% in the 30 minutes after the subject had smoked two cigarettes. Injections of nicotine also increased dogs' cholesterol levels by 34% and decreased the flow of blood in the coronary vessels. By blocking the release of free fatty acids, niacin prevents one of the health-damaging cycles related to smoking.

Stroke

Strokes are largely preventable if certain risk factors are avoided. Niacin, by correcting lipid profiles, reduces a major risk factor.

Dr Hoffer has studied the effect of niacin on his patients who had already suffered brain damage from stroke or trauma. He became interested after reading a report from Sweden many years ago about the treatment of strokes. The authors reported that stroke patients on admission to hospital were promptly given IV niacin and, as a result, experienced a marked reduction in the incidence of subsequent strokes. McCracken also referred to a Norwegian study where arteries leading to a dog's heart were tied, thus simulating a heart attack.[14] Giving intravenous niacin 15 minutes after the restriction and continuing it for 30 minutes decreased the heart damage.

Among patients in Dr Hoffer's care, C.B., a middle-aged woman who had prided herself on her memory, had a mild stroke, but after her recovery, her memory was not nearly as good. She found this a terrible handicap. After a few months on niacin, her memory was partially restored and she was content.

Another case involved a young man who was struck on the head by a heavy object during an industrial accident. After 2 years, he was able to talk and to walk with a limp, but he had not regained his interest in reading. Before the accident he had been an avid reader. After 3 months on niacin, he regained some of this interest and became content with this improvement.

Apparently, niacin, by dilating the capillaries, accelerated healing and perhaps also increased the ability of the brain tissue to repair itself. Such repair has always been considered impossible, but as medicine progresses, the formerly impossible often becomes commonplace.

Indeed, evidence is accumulating that niacin helps recovery of the damaged brain. J. Yang and coworkers, for example, found that nicotinamide could rescue viable but injured nerve cells within the ischemic area after experimental strokes in animals.[15] Early injection of nicotinamide reduced the number of necrotic and apoptotic neurons. Later injections were not as effective. Yang and Adams concluded that "early administration of nicotinamide may be of therapeutic interest in preventing the development of stroke, by rescuing the still viable but injured nerve cells and partially preventing infarction."[16]

They also found that vitamin B-3 decreased the progression of neurodegenerative disease. It prevented learning and memory impairment caused by cerebral oxidative stress. According to these studies, nicoti-namide works more quickly than niacin, but both are inter-convertible, though niacin will likely have an advantage because it dilates the capillar-ies. In addition, C.W. Levenson has reviewed the findings that with trau-matic brain injury, zinc is released.[17] Accumulation of high amounts of free zinc leads to the loss of NAD. Supplements of vitamin B-3 increase NAD levels.

Atrial Fibrillation

In combination with folic acid, niacin has been shown to be therapeutic against atrial fibrillation, as seen among several patients in Dr Hoffer's care. The first case was a physician, age 70, who had been on nicotinic acid for many years, 3 to 6 g daily. On this dose, he developed lymphedema in the left leg. In an effort to deal with this problem, he discontinued his nicotinic acid. The edema cleared, but, after many months, he began to suffer a number of disturbing symptoms, including a very low pulse rate, which was not responsive to demand, remaining slow even when he tried to walk fast, and would begin to speed up only after a few minutes. He became very short of breath and suffered episodes of tachycardia (the sudden racing of the heart), which were controlled by pressure on the carotids in his neck or by changes in body position. Such rapid heart beat episodes lasted up to 20 minutes and were accompanied by shortness of breath and sometimes dizziness.

On physical examination, he was normal, as was his electrocardiogram, and he had a normal sinus rhythm. He resumed taking the nicotinic acid, starting with a low dose and gradually working up to 4.5 g daily. At the same time, he increased his folic acid from the 5 mg he had been taking daily for several years to 40 mg daily. He continued to take daily vitamin B-12, 1 mg sublingually. By the time these dosage levels were reached, after a couple of months all the heart rate symptoms vanished. He can now walk with no shortness of breath.

The second case of atrial fibrillation involved a physician aged 76. She had consulted Dr Hoffer for advice in treating a young patient, who sub-sequently recovered on vitamin B-3 and vitamin C. This physician was so impressed with this patient's recovery that she had decided to place herself on a vitamin program. This regimen included 1 g of niacin and 15 mg of folic acid twice a day. During one of her visits, she described how she had suffered periods of atrial fibrillation lasting for as long as 3 hours at a time, before starting on the vitamins. Only when she went off the program for several months did it recur.

A third patient, age 72, consulted Dr Hoffer for severe depression. In 1981, she had a coronary. She was advised she would suffer pain after this and she did. In 1988, she was admitted to hospital for severe chest pain. Thereafter, she had recurrent painful episodes every 3 weeks, unrelated to activity or exertion. In 1989, she was in hospital for 1 week for depression. She then started on niacin 500 mg, three times a day, together with doses of antidepressants. She recovered and remained well until April 1993. She was then admitted to hospital with atrial fibrillation.

In June 1993, her pulse rate was around 100. Dr Hoffer added 5 mg of folic acid, three times a day, to her program. She remained on digoxin. By March 1994, she was well. She had very few brief episodes of pain, no fibrillation, and was able to walk 1.5 miles daily and to garden with no difficulty.

Nephritis

L. Condorelli reported that 20 years of experience with nicotinic acid had confirmed its efficacy in acute diffuse glomerulonephritis. He established that in sub-acute or chronic forms and in other nephritic disorders this treatment may also beneficial.[18] Two patients in Dr Hoffer's care with nephritis have been cured by niacin.

When A.W. first visited Dr Hoffer, she explained that her nephrologist had told her that that she had severe nephritis and that she would need a kidney transplant. She was advised to return to her nephrologist with copies of Dr Condorelli's studies on niacin. Twenty years later, Dr Hoffer had dinner with her in Victoria and was reminded by her husband of this event. She then described how she had discussed niacin with her nephrologist, who laughed at her, but she became more determined than ever that she would not have a transplant and instead began to take niacin on her own. She has been well since.

The second case was a 12-year-old girl who had severe acute nephrites, for which she was advised there was no treatment. Her father, a highschool teacher, began to read as much as he could on the illness and, on his own, started her on niacin. She recovered and then visited Dr Max Vogel, who confirmed her former illness and recovery from it.

References

[1] Public Health Agency of Canada. Heart Disease and Stroke in Canada 1997. http://www.phac-aspc.gc.ca/publicat/hdsc97/s02°e.html

[2] Public Health Agency of Canada. Heart Disease and Stroke in Canada 1997. http://www.phac-aspc.gc.ca/publicat/hdsc97/s02°e.html

[3] bmj.com Letters. Why heart disease mortality is low in France. http://bmj.bmjjournals.com/cgi/content/full/319/7204/255

[4] Department of Health. Coronary Heart Disease. http://www.dh.gov.uk/PolicyAndGuidance/HealthAndSocialCareTopics/CoronaryHeartDisease/fs/en

[5] Condorelli L. Nicotinic acid in the therapy of the cardiovascular apparatus. In: Niacin in Vascular Disorders and Hyperlipemia. Altschul R (ed.). Springfield, IL: CC Thomas, 1964.

[6] McCracken RD. Niacin and Human Health Disorders. Fort Collins, CO: Hygea Publishing Co., 1994.

[7] Altschul R, Hoffer A, Stephen JD. Influence of nicotinic acid on serum cholesterol in man. *Arch Biochem Biophys.* 1955;54:558-59.

[8] Parsons WB Jr. Cholesterol Control without Diet! The Niacin Solution. Revised, Expanded, 2nd ed. Scottsdale, AZ: Lilac Press, 2003.

[9] Canner PL, Berge KG, Wenger NK, et al. Fifteen-year Mortality in Coronary Drug Project Patients; Long-tern Benefit with Niacin. *J Am Col Cardiology* 1986;8:1245-55.

[10] Brown B Greg, Zhao X, Chait A, et al. Simvastatin and niacin, antioxidant vitamins, or the combination for the prevention of coronary disease. *New England Journal of Medicine* 2001;345:1583-92.

[11] McKenney J. New perspectives on the use of niacin in the treatment of lipid disorders. *Archives Internal Medicine* 2004;164:697-704.

[12] Munro M. Cholesterol pill's side effects worry BC drug specialists. Victoria, BC: Times-Colonist, September 16, 2003.

13 Graveline D. Transient global amnesia. A side effect of "statins" treatment. Townsend Letter for Doctors and Patients 2004 Aug/Sept;253/254:85-89.

14 McCracken RD. Niacin and Human Health Disorders. Fort Collins, Colorado: Hygea Publishing Co., 1994.

15 Yang J, Klaidman LK, Adams JD. Medicinal chemistry of nicotinamide in the treatment of ischemia and reperfusion. Mini Reviews in Medicinal Chemistry 2002;2:125-34.

16 Yang J, Adams JD. Nicotinamide and its pharmacological properties for clinical therapy. Drug Design Reviews 2004;1:43-52.

17 Levenson CW. Zinc Supplementation: Neuroprotective or neurotoxic? Nutrition Reviews 2005;63:122-25.

18 Condorelli L. Nicotinic acid in the therapy of the cardiovascular apparatus. In: Niacin in Vascular Disorders and Hyperlipemia. Altschul R (ed.). Springfield, IL: CC Thomas, 1964.

HUNTINGTON'S DISEASE

Prevalence

Huntington's disease is a rare inherited neurological disorder that affects 1 out of 20,000 people of Western European descent and only 7 in one million of Asian or African descent. In Canada, 2.14 people die from it per million people in the population. It is strongly genetic. Half of the children of a parent who carries the gene will also develop the disease, with symptoms usually starting between ages 35 and 44. There are no periods of remission. About 70% of patients with Huntington's disease die within 15 years of its onset.

Role of Vitamin B-3

This devastating illness is characterized by both mental and physical symptoms. The physical symptoms are very similar to those found in Parkinson's Disease, but also include severe and dangerous weight loss. The mental symptoms are similar to schizophrenia, and they appear before physical symptoms.

Dr Charles N. Still has argued that Huntington's disease and pellagra are very similar clinically.[1,2] He concluded that pellagra was a good clinical model for Huntington's disease. Huntington's is considered to be one of the schizophrenic syndromes, amenable to treatment with vitamin B-3.

Clinical Evidence

In 1973, a 60-year old man came limping into Dr Hoffer's office, accompanied by his wife. She said he had Huntington's disease. Although Hoffer explained he was not familiar with the disease and there was no known treatment, she replied that they wanted to try an orthomolecular approach.

The patient's father and uncle had previously died psychotic in a mental hospital with the disease. There were five male siblings in the family. The oldest was in a nursing home, bedridden and psychotic, and the youngest brother had also been placed in a nursing home, where he died 1 year after admission.

The patient's symptoms began when he was 40 and gradually became worse. His original weight had been 165 lbs, but had fallen to 130 lbs due to muscle tissue loss. He was so weak that it took all his energy just to survive: to eat, dress, and look after himself. He was tired all the time. He walked with a jerky limp. He had no hallucinations, but his cognition was affected. He could not think clearly, his memory was faulty, and he was depressed, anxious, and tense. He had been advised that he probably could not be helped in order not to generate unwarranted hope.

Dr Hoffer advised him to start a low-sugar, junk-free diet and added B vitamins and vitamin C. After 1 month he was not as depressed, his concentration was better, and he was able to work for the first time in many years. Two months later, he was still free of depression. By this time, he was taking 3 g of niacin daily, 1.5 g of vitamin C daily, and a megavitamin containing B-1 (100 mg), B-2 (25 mg), B-6 (25 mg), and niacinamide (100 mg). He was also receiving a weekly B-12 injection (1 mg) and folic acid, 5 mg twice daily. At 2 months, vitamin E (400 IU, twice daily) was added.

Six months after he was first seen, his weight had fallen to 125 lbs. Because he was still losing weight, which was ominous, his vitamin E intake was increased to 800 IU, twice daily. This stabilized his weight, and after another month, he gained 2 lbs. After 11 months, he was back to 135 lbs. His muscles were recovering their bulk and strength. His chest, which had been collapsing, was back to normal. At this point, the vitamin E was again increased to 1,600 IU, twice daily. After 13 months, he weighed 139 lbs.

His niacin was decreased to 500 mg after each meal and eventually replaced with an equal amount of niacinamide. At 17 months, he was as well as he had been before he first became sick. At 22 months, he stopped the niacinamide to see if he still needed it, but within a few weeks, he became very restless and tense, and his legs stiffened when he walked. Back on niacinamide, he was normal in a few days. Three years later when last seen, he was well.

The most impressive response came from the vitamin B-3 and from the vitamin E. Only after the addition of a large dose of vitamin E did the muscular deterioration stop, while vitamin B-3 restored his brain function. When he stopped taking this vitamin for a few days, his condition recurred. He apparently had a double vitamin dependency, on vitamin B-3 for the psychiatric component of his illness, and on vitamin E for its physical dimensions. Huntington's disease, therefore, may be a double dependency disease.

Dr Hoffer was involved with a second such patient, who was not seen but who kept him informed of his progress. In 1978, A.K. wrote to Dr Hoffer and described his recovery from schizophrenia on niacin. He had been treated by Dr Hitchings in New York after jumping out of a third-story window and breaking his back during a psychotic episode. He subsequently made a complete mental recovery. However, his wife, an engineer, could not work because she was too tired. Excessive fatigue is one of the early symptoms of Huntington's disease. Her mother was psychotic in a French mental hospital, and she was very concerned about the possibility of transmitting this illness to her children. She wondered if niacin, which had cured her husband, might it not also help her.

She was advised that the vitamin program was safe, and she began to take vitamin E (800 IU), niacin (1.5 g), vitamin C (1 g), and one multiple vitamin tablet. Three years later, she was well, and although she had been unable to work for the previous 7 years because of gross fatigue, she was now employed. The perceptual illusions that had prevented her from driving a car were gone. So, too, were her fears and memory problems. Her husband, a well known poet, wrote that "the change in [B.K.] since she started the vitamin treatment and particularly the choline has been nothing short of amazing."

For the treatment of Huntington's disease, high dose vitamin B-3, vitamin E, and other vitamins, as well as adequate nutrition, with up to 5,000 calories daily given in five meals, is recommended.

References

[1] Still CN. Nutritional therapy in Huntingtons's chorea: Concepts based on the model of pellagra. Psychiatric Forum 1979;9:74-78.

[2] Still CN. Sex differences affecting nutritional therapy in Huntington's disease: An inherited essential fatty acid metabolic disorder. Psychiatric Forum 1980-1981;9:47-51.

PARKINSON'S DISEASE

Prevalence

There are marked international, national, and local spatial variations in the incidence and prevalence of Parkinson's disease, suggesting that the environment or lifestyle play a key role in its etiology. It is rare under age 50. The estimated annual cost of treating such patients in Canada is $500 million, while average monthly drug costs are some $1,000. About 24,000 to 39,000 Canadians have Parkinson's disease. In the United States about 1 in 200 of the population suffer from this disease, although it is most common in Afro-Americans.

Role of L-dopa

There was no effective treatment for Parkinson's disease until it was discovered that L-dopa ameliorated its symptoms. Initially, a double-blind clinical study indicated that L-dopa was not effective, but the dose range used was inadequate and, subsequently, more appropriate levels exhibited its efficacy.[1,2]

This discovery supported the hypothesis that, in Parkinson's disease, not enough dopamine was available to the brain. L-dopa, of course, increased the amount of this amine. Unfortunately, this was a mixed blessing because patients on L-dopa could easily become psychotic and have reduced life expectancy if too much was prescribed. Adrenal gland grafts can also trigger psychosis. Interestingly, both L-dopa and adrenal grafts increase the amount of brain dopamine, but, in Parkinson's disease, this may be oxidized to dopachrome and similar toxic compounds, especially in the absence of adequate natural anti-oxidants.

Dr Hoffer and Dr Foster have discussed such psychotomimetic effects of L-dopa in an article published in *Medical Hypotheses*.[3] These effects have also been highlighted by Dr Oliver Sacks, who described the remarkable effect of L-dopa on patients with *Encephalitis lethargica*, as dramatized in the film *Awakenings*.[4,5] Sacks treated 20 such patients, starting with 500 mg of L-dopa daily, but increasing it, if required, to 6 g. Many of his patients showed great early progress, but this was not sustained. They all reverted back to their original state and quickly died. Such huge doses of L-dopa are certainly very toxic to the brain.

Role of Vitamin B-3

D r Hoffer has discovered that high doses of niacin are very helpful in preventing Parkinson's psychosis. His use of this vitamin is based on the adrenochrome hypothesis of schizophrenia, described previously.

As described in *Medical Hypotheses*,[6] three measures must be addressed when treating Parkinson's disease:

- Deal with oxidative stress (decreasing it where possible) by using natural anti-oxidants
- Give natural methyl acceptors (the most readily available of which is vitamin B-3)
- Use high dose anti-oxidants to mitigate the adverse toxic effects of L-dopa

Clinical Evidence

I n 1993, J.G.D. Birkmayer and coworkers found that both oral and parenteral NADH were equally effective in Parkinson's disease.[7] They treated

885 patients with one or other of these methods and found that only about 20% did not benefit. Younger patients, who had not been symptomatic as long, responded better. To avoid damage in the stomach, their oral preparation had to be stabilized. NADH in ordinary gelatin capsules was not effective, as had been found with NAD when treating schizophrenic patients.

About 10 years ago, after it was reported that brain cells of Parkinson's patients were also deficient in coenzyme Q10, Dr Hoffer added this antioxidant to his treatment protocol. In addition to the niacin and other nutrients they were taking, his Parkinson's patients were given coenzyme Q10, 600 mg daily, for 2 weeks, which was then decreased to 300 mg. They were all also on L-dopa. To date, they have all remained mentally normal, probably because of their high dose of niacin. Fortunately, their physical symptoms have improved substantially and stabilized.

Coenzyme Q10 is now well established as part of the treatment for Parkinson's disease, as shown in several recent studies. According to research conducted by K. Winkler-Stuck and colleagues, there is a generalized deficiency in the mitochondria that can be ameliorated by coenzyme Q10.[8] H.R. Larsen has also discussed the importance of anti-oxidants in Parkinson's disease treatment.[9] Shultz and coworkers have found that 1200 mg per day of coenzyme Q10 is more therapeutic than lower doses.[10] However, they were not treating their patients with niacin and other anti-oxidants. If these anti-oxidants had been given long before the first significant symptoms of Parkinson's disease occurred, they might have been prevented in the majority of cases.

References

[1] Foley P. The L-DOPA story revisited. Further surprises to be expected. J Neural Transm Suppl 2000;60:1-20.

[2] Cotzias GC, Van Woert MH, Schiffer LM. Aromatic amino acids and modification of Parkinsonism. N Engl J Med 1967;276(7):374-379.

[3] Foster HD, Hoffer A. The two faces of L-dopa: Benefits and adverse side effects in the treatment of Encephalitis lethargica, Parkinson's disease, multiple sclerosis and amyotrophic lateral sclerosis. Medical Hypotheses 2004;62:177-81.

4 Sacks O. The origin of "Awakenings." Br Med J (Clin Res Ed). 1983;287(6409):1968-1969.

5 Columbia Pictures Corporation. Zaillian S (Screenplay). Awakenings; 1990.

6 Foster HD, Hoffer A. The two faces of L-dopa: Benefits and adverse side effects in the treatment of Encephalitis lethargica, Parkinson's disease, multiple sclerosis and amyotrophic lateral sclerosis. Medical Hypotheses 2004;62:177-81.

7 Birkmayer JGD, Vrecko C, Volc D, Birkmayer W. Nicotinamide adenine dinucleotide (NADH): A new therapeutic approach to Parkinson's disease. Comparison of oral and parenteral application. Acta Neurol Scand 1993;87:32-35

8 Winkler-Stuck K, Wiedermann FR, Wallesh CW, Kunz WS. Effect of coenzyme Q 10 on the mitochondrial function of skin fibroblasts from Parkinson's patients. J Neurol Sci 2004;220:41-44.

9 Larsen HR. Parkinson's disease: Is victory in sight? International Journal of Alternative and Complementary Medicine 1997;15:22-24.

10 Shults CW, Oakes D, Kieburtz K, Beal MF, Haas R, Plumb S et al. Parkinson Study Group. Effects of Coenzyme Q10 in early Parkinson's disease: Evidence of slowing of functional decline. Arch Neurol. 2002;59(10):1541-1550.

ARTHRITIS

Prevalence

The 2000 Canadian Community Health Survey (CCHS) established that arthritis and other rheumatoid conditions affected approximately one Canadian in six. Two-thirds of those suffering from arthritis were women, and nearly three out of five of those suffering from it were younger than 65 years old.[1] In the United States, arthritis and other rheumatic conditions are costing approximately $128 billion annually, about 1.2% of the gross domestic product.[2] The United States prevalence rate for self-referred arthritis is expected to rise from 15% of the population in 1990 to 18.2% by 2020. This figure will represent 59.4 million cases.[3]

Role of Vitamin B-3

In the 1940s, Dr William Kaufman was the first to report that niacinamide in large doses, starting from 250 mg, taken four times daily, was useful in reversing the changes normally associated with old age.[4,5] His primary interest was in reversing arthritic symptoms, but he observed significant associated improvement in other functions.

A few months after the first report by Dr Hoffer and colleagues was published on the therapeutic effect of vitamin B-3 on schizophrenic patients in 1957, Dr Kaufman responded that they were wrong in claiming they were the first to use large doses of this vitamin therapeutically. "Ever since 1943," he wrote, "I have tried to call my work on niacinamide to the attention of leading hematologists, nutritionists and gerontologists through conversations with them, by sending them copies of my monograph and paper on this subject and by two talks on the usefulness of niacinamide and other vitamins, which I gave at International Gerontological Congresses in 1951 and 1954. I think two factors have made it difficult for doctors to accept the concept that continuous therapy with large doses of niacinamide could cause improvement to joint dysfunction and give other benefits: (a) the advent of cortisone and (b) the fact that my use of the vitamins was such a departure from the recommended daily allowance for vitamins by the National Research Council."[6] Subsequent research has shown that vitamin B-3 is, in fact, effective for treating osteoarthritis and rheumatoid arthritis.

Clinical Evidence

In 1954, Dr Hoffer was awarded a Rockefeller Fellow Travel Grant to study European psychiatric research. Before leaving for Europe, Dr Hoffer, his wife Rose, and Bill, his 10-year old son, visited his parents. Dr Hoffer's mother, then 67 years old, was not well. Her health problems included an inability to see from her left eye, painful arthritis in both hands, tiredness, and generally feeling unwell. As a standard physician, Dr Hoffer 'knew' that these were all old age changes and that there was nothing anyone could do about it. However, as a psychiatrist he also 'knew' that he should offer some hope; provide her with a placebo, if nothing else. By this time he had several years experience taking niacin and niacinamide. They were safe. He also felt that the initial flushing would give greater credibility to the placebo and could not do his mother any harm.

At his urging, his mother agreed to take 1 g of niacin, three times daily after meals. Soon after, Dr Hoffer and his family sailed to England. About 1 month later, a letter arrived at Saskatchewan House in London from his mother. She wrote that she was very much better: she could see again clearly and the arthritis was leaving her hands. "Those little bumps were going away." Dr Hoffer was delighted, but suspected that none of this could be true because those little bumps (Heberdens nodes) never went away. When he visited his mother upon returning from Europe 3 months later, he discovered that she was indeed very much better. Her mind was clear and the arthritic nodes were flattening out. Dr Hoffer's mother remained well on high dose niacin until she died in 1975, age 88. During the last few years of her life, she completed two books describing her early experiences living in southern Saskatchewan.

A second member of the Hoffer family also benefited from the niacin 'placebo'. Dr Hoffer's father-in-law developed arthritis and gout. The gout was easily treated by his doctors, but they did not have the same luck with his arthritis. Dr Hoffer advised him to try high dose niacin, and he responded very well. Although his arthritis cleared, his gout continued to come and go as before. Niacin apparently had no effect on it, neither making it worse nor better.

Dr Hoffer then prepared a brief report of his work, supported by the results of six cases.[7] One patient with osteoarthritis became normal, another with rheumatoid arthritis became much better. Two other arthritis cases became normal, while one patient with both schizophrenia and arthritis became completely well. The last, who suffered from vascular nodulitis, was much improved.

Since then, many of Dr Hoffer's patients with arthritis have recovered or become much better when prescribed niacin. The most dramatic case came into his office in a wheelchair, pushed by her very tired and sick-looking husband. She was sitting with her legs crossed over as she could not extend them. She had been sick for the previous 20 years and had tried every known treatment for arthritis, including hormone and gold injections. Nothing had helped. Her hands were totally useless; she was crippled. Her husband had to carry her around the house, even to the bathroom. He provided her with the equivalent care of four nurses, around the clock. No wonder he was totally exhausted and looking ill.

Because very chronic deteriorated arthritis cases generally did not do well, Dr Hoffer offered little hope for recovery. But this patient persisted: "I know that you cannot help my arthritis, but the pain in my back is terrible. All I want is some relief from it." She was started on a vitamin program, with niacin as the main constituent. This patient returned a month later in her wheelchair, again being pushed by her husband. This time, however, she was sitting in her chair with her feet dangling straight down. Her husband looked relaxed and had lost his dreadful sick look. When Dr Hoffer began to talk, she interrupted and said, "The pain is gone." She was so improved that Hoffer began to think that maybe, with skillful surgery, some function might be restored to her hands.

Six months later she telephoned Dr Hoffer, who asked her in surprise, "How did you get to the phone?" She replied that she was now able to get around on her own in her chair. However, she was not calling for herself, but for her husband who had a cold. She wanted some advice about how to help him. This woman died several years later, having achieved her goal of a pain-free existence.

In 1999, Dan Lukaczer in *Nutrition Science* reported confirmation of Dr William Kaufman's pioneering research in treating arthritis with vitamin B-3.[8] "A few years ago," he wrote, "Wayne Jonas from the NIH Office of Alternative Medicine in Bethesda, MD, conducted a 12-week, double-blind, placebo-controlled study of 72 patients to assess the validity of Kaufman's earlier observations that niacin was of great benefit to the elderly, reducing arthritis. Jonas reported that niacinamide at 3 g/day reduced overall disease severity by 29%, inflammation by 22% and use of anti-inflammatory medication by 13%." [9] Patients in the placebo group either had no improvement or worsened.

Although these may be considered only modest changes, Kaufman had emphasized that improvement among his patients started after 4 to 12 weeks – the time at which Jonas' study stopped. He also found that people might continue to improve for up to a year before they plateaued. Jonas' study identified no significant side effects, but to be safe, those who opt for long-term niacinamide therapy should have their liver enzymes periodically assessed by a doctor.

Arthritis has recently been at the center of a vortex of medical controversy. In October 2004, Vioxx, one of the main drugs used to treat arthritis, was voluntarily withdrawn by its manufacturers, Merck and Co. Some 70,000 deaths, largely from cardiovascular episodes, had been associated with this drug's use. Such toxic side effects had been known by the industry for several years. In February 2005, a panel of the U.S. Food and Drug

Administration voted to allow the possible return of Vioxx, provided it carried a striking black-box warning on its label about its cardiovascular risks. Patients who take it will be obliged to sign consent forms.

Interestingly, the *Globe and Mail* reported that 10 of the 32 members of the U.S. Food and Drug Administration panel voting to allow the return of Vioxx had worked as consultants, in recent years, for the drug's makers.[10] This panel also supported the continued use of other cox-2 drugs, such as Celebrex and Bextra, for arthritis, despite their known cardiovascular risks, so long as they also carry a black-box warning. Given the evidence that arthritis can often be successfully treated with vitamins B-3 and C or other nutrients, these decisions raise many interesting ethical issues.

Vitamin B-3 is not a drug. Drugs are developed to treat a single condition. Arthritis is not a single disease. It is caused by many factors, including toxic responses to foods. Reactions to dairy foods and nightshades (potato, tomato, egg plant), for example, can cause arthritis. Other vitamin and mineral deficiencies may also be involved, including pyridoxine and zinc deficiencies. Factors such as chronic infections also have to be considered. Vitamin B-3 is important in the treatment of arthritis, but there are other significant therapeutic substances and strategies.

References

[1] Health Canada. Arthritis in Canada. An Ongoing Challenge. Ottawa: Health Canada, 2003.

[2] National Center for Chronic Disease Prevention and Health Promotion. Arthritis Data and Statistics. http://www.cdc.gov/arthritis/data°statistics/cost°data.htm

[3] Centers for Disease Control and Prevention. Arthritis Prevalence and Activity Limitations – United States, 1990. Morbidity and Mortality Weekly Report 1994; 43(24):433-438.

[4] Kaufman W. Common Forms of Niacinamide Deficiency Disease: Aniacin Amidosis. New Haven, CT: Yale University Press, 1943.

[5] Kaufman W. The Common Form of Joint Dysfunction: Its Incidence and Treatment. Brattleboro, CT: EL Hildreth and Co, 1949.

6 Kaufman W. Niacinamide: A most neglected vitamin. J Int Acad Preventvie Medicine.1983;8:5-25.

7 Hoffer A. Treatment of arthritis by nicotinic acid and nicotinamide. Can Med Ass J 1959; 81:235-38.

8 Lukaczer D. Nutrition Q and A. Nutrition Science News. November 1999. http://www.newhope.com/nutritionsciencenews/NSN°backs/Nov°99/q°and°a.cfm

9 Jonas WB, Rapoza CP, Blair WF. The effect of niacinamide on osteoarthritis: A pilot study. Inflamm Res 1996;45:330-34.

10 Abraham C. Vioxx makers 'perplexed' by Dosanjh's remarks. Today's Paper Health. http://www.theglobeandmail.com/servlet/ArticleNews/TPStory/LAC/20050226/Vioxx26/TPHealth/

ALZHEIMER'S DISEASE AND SENILITY

Prevalence

As Dr Foster has described in his book, *What Really Causes Alzheimer's Disease*, this illness is increasing because life expectancies have risen significcantly during the past century.[1] As a consequence, in both the developed and developing world, the number of elderly has undergone an unprecedented increase, with the proportion of the very old in the population doubling in one generation. Globally, in 1950 there were 214 million people aged 60 or more; by 2025 there probably will be one billion, a more than four-fold increase.[2]

Although there are major advantages associated with this trend, there are also serious costs. Not only are more people surviving into old age and, therefore, increasing their chances of developing dementia, but those who do so are living longer after its onset. In the United States, for example, Alzheimer's disease prevalence, currently affecting approximately 4.5 million people, is expected to increase by 350% by mid-century to 14 million, clustering in those states with the highest numbers of retired baby boomers.[3] It is predicted that by 2025, 820,000 elderly Californians,

712,000 Floridians, and 552,000 Texans will be suffering from Alzheimer's disease.[4] The high costs of caring for these millions of demented elderly may wreak havoc on the healthcare system.

This paradox has been called the "failure of success" because it was a major problem that was largely attributable to progress in medical care.[5] As E.M. Gruenberg and his colleagues point out, "the old man's friend, pneumonia, is dead – a victim of medical progress."[6] While this is an over-simplification, pneumonia is certainly less common than it used to be, as are many other diseases that were previously fatal to the elderly.

It has been estimated that approximately eight million people in the European Union member states in 2000 had Alzheimer's disease. Since this disorder accounts for about 50% of all dementia in people over 65, total esti-mates for dementia in Europe are closer to 16 million. As in North America, the European population is aging rapidly and the number of senile demen-tia cases is increasing accordingly.[7] Clearly, in the Western World, dementia is not a rare problem. Indeed, R. Katzman and colleagues have argued that in people more than 75 years of age, new cases of dementia occur as fre-quently as myocardial infarction and twice as often as stroke.[8]

Role of Vitamin B-3

Since 1955, Dr Hoffer has given his patients niacin when they have symp-toms of senility (premature aging).[9,10] It is most helpful in the early stages of senility, especially if patients have a history of cardiovascular prob-lems or if their cholesterol levels are elevated. It is of little benefit when senility is fully developed. Another beneficial effect of niacin is that it diminishes or removes xanthomatous deposits and fat deposits in the skin.

There appears to be a statistically significant link between a low dietary intake of niacin and a high risk of developing Alzheimer's disease. M.C. Morris and coworkers, for example, conducted a prospective study of the niacin intake of 6,158 Chicago residents 65 years of age or older.[11] This established that the lower the daily intake of niacin, the greater the risk of becoming an Alzheimer's disease patient. Specifically, the quintile with the highest mean daily intake (45 mg) had a 70% decrease in incidence of this disease compared to the quintile with the lowest mean daily niacin con-sumption (14 mg).

Alzheimer's disease has traditionally been considered untreatable, except by a few drugs, which, at best, may slow the degenerative process a little. Niacin does not help fully developed Alzheimer's disease either, but there is growing evidence that this disease can be prevented by the proper use of nutrients. Professor Foster, for example, has argued at length that this disease is caused by an excess of monomeric aluminum in people who are calcium and magnesium deficient.[12]

Clinical Evidence

In 1962, Dr Hoffer reported that senility is a form of chronic malnutrition, a nutrient deficiency disorder that can be improved or even reversed with large doses of vitamin B-3 and other nutrients.[13, 14] "There seems to be no reason why old people should develop the type of intellectual and mental deterioration found in senile states," he argued. "Indeed, the brain is exposed to so little mechanical wear and tear that it ought to be the last organ in the body to deteriorate. For apart from the gentle pulsations of the blood vessels, the even gentler contraction and expansions of the neuroglia, it has achieved a state of perfection in which its essential activity is the transmission of ions (electrical impulses). These functions are surely less harmful to tissues than the attrition of bone upon bone at the joints, for example. Heart, muscle, bones, joints, skin and the hollow viscera, which move continuously or act as bearings, must all, one would suppose, be subjected to continuous mechanical deterioration due to friction and flexion. These organs ought to deteriorate long before the brain does... All that has to be done is (1) to reduce the small amount of vascular wear and tear in the brain, and (2) discover and then inhibit chemical changes in cerebral tissues which lead to tissue failure."

Hoffer reviewed the early literature that showed niacin, thiamin, and liver extract inhibited senility from developing and described senile patients from his practice who were treated with niacin. Their mean age was 69. Five senile psychotics recovered. Two were markedly improved by niacin, and two were not helped by it. Six were depressed, not senile, and of these, five recovered and remained well.

The best results were seen when the niacin was given before definite senile changes occurred. It has been shown that mean IQ decreases with age in a linear manner, dropping from 110 at age 30 to 70 at age 79.5. It would seem that the best time to counter senility with niacin is between 30 and 60 years of age. In the book *Smart Nutrients: Prevent and Treat Alzheimer's and Senility, Enhance Brain Function and Longevity*, co-authored by Dr Abram Hoffer and Dr Morton Walker, these findings are elaborated and corroborated with additional clinical evidence showing the therapeutic effect of vitamin B-3 as an anti-aging agent.

Niacin is known to lower total cholesterol, LDL, and triglycerides, while elevating HDL. Perhaps these characteristics are what gives niacin its anti-aging properties, recently confirmed by the Women's Health Study presented at the Ninth International Conference on Alzheimer's Disease.[15] Beginning in 1991, nearly 40,000 women 66 years of age or older were enrolled in this study, which established that those in the highest HDL quintile had the least chance of developing cognitive impairment. Although there was no association shown with other lipids, a linearly decreasing risk was associated with increasing levels of HDL. Women in the highest quintile had only one-fifth the chance of developing Alzheimer's disease as those in the lowest quintile. Niacin is the best substance that is known to elevate HDL.

Vitamin B-3 is a superior to aspirin as anti-aging agent. Aspirin used in low dose is widely touted as the one of the main answers to geriatric decline, but it has serious side-effects, such as excessive bleeding. It is estimated that 67 patients must take aspirin in order to protect one against a stroke or myocardial infarction, but from each 100, one will suffer serious bleeding. In comparison, niacin is safe. However, it is not easy to compare niacin and aspirin since no one has estimated the likely long-term effects of niacin in the same way that those of aspirin and the statins have been examined. Niacin cannot be patented, and, as a result, no company can profit from such a study.[16, 17]

It is not suggested here that niacin alone is the answer to preventing Alzheimer's disease. Indeed, the most compelling evidence to date is that early memory loss can be reversed by the ascorbate minerals.[18-20] Greater Alzheimer's disease risk also has been linked to low dietary intake of vitamin E and of fish.[21-24] The elderly should continue to eat well balanced diets, high in calcium, magnesium, selenium, the B vitamins, and essential fatty acids. Aluminum, especially in its monomeric form, should be avoided. Niacin supplements are recommended as a precaution.

Dr Roger Williams, the great biochemist who discovered both folic and pantothenic acids, has commented, "every kind of essential nutrient comes into play in the promotion and prolongation of healthy life." Credit for longevity must also be given to other factors, including genes. But our 'longevity genes' function best when the body is provided with vitamin B-3 (nicotinic acid and or nicotinamide or nicotinamide adenine dinucleotide), as well as anti-oxidant vitamins and minerals, and protected from toxic metals and xenobiotic chemicals.

Dr Williams died when he was 95 years of age. Toward the end of his life, he was nearly totally deaf and blind, but his mind was as sharp as ever. Dr Williams confided in Dr Hoffer that he was very sorry he had not started taking vitamins early in his life. He was sure that they would have prevented both of his major infirmities.

Dr Williams is not the only orthomolecular doctor to have lived a long and productive life. The first members of the new Orthomolecular Medicine Hall of Fame were announced in 2004. Listed below are these members together with their ages and their main areas of interest nutritionally. On average, they lived for 84.1 years and, in contrast to most men, their productivity did not decrease with age. On the contrary, it increased.

Linus Pauling	1901 to 1994	vitamin C
William McCormick	1880 to 1968	vitamin C
Roger J. Williams	1893 to 1988	folate, pantothenate
Wilfred Shute	1907 to 1982	alpha tocopherol
Evan Shute	1905 to 1978	alpha tocopherol
Irwin Stone	1907 to 1984	vitamin C
Carl C. Pfeiffer	1908 to 1988	B vitamins and C
Allan Cott	1910 to 1993	niacin
William Kaufman	1910 to 2000	nicotinamide
Humphry Osmond	1917 to 2004	niacin and vitamin C

The 2005 inductees in to the Hall of Fame lived on average for 82 years.

Max Gerson	1881 to 1959	nutrition and niacin
Albert Szent-Gyorgi	1893 to 1986	vitamin C
Cornelius Moerman	1893 to 1988	nutrition and B vitamins

Frederick Klenner	1907 to 1984	high dose vitamin C
Josef Issels	1907 to 1998	nutrition
Emanuel Cheraskin	1916 to 2001	nutrition and vitamins
David Horrobin	1939 to 2003	essential fatty acids
Hugh Desaix Riordan	1932 to 2005	nutrition and vitamins

Dr Hoffer had a female patient who died at 112 years of age. She had been well, both physically and mentally, until shortly before her death. She was the oldest person in the Province of Saskatchewan, and was still cross country skiing when she was 109 years old. This woman had been taking elevated niacin for 41 years. She was photographed playing a piano duet with her great grandson shortly before she died.[25] Dr Hoffer himself is in his 90th year.

In *Smart Nutrients*, Hoffer and Walker wrote, "it has been said that old age can become an expression of human experience. It can be rich, varied, colorful, and in turn enriching; or it can be impoverished, empty, and only serve to emphasize the futility of life." [26] For the elderly today, reality is too often the latter possibility, but the use of therapeutic levels of vitamin B-3 and other nutrients can make the former possibility a reality.

References

[1] Foster HD. What Really Causes Alzheimer's Disease. Victoria, BC: Trafford Publishing, 2004.

[2] Henderson AS. The epidemiology of Alzheimer's disease. British Medical Bulletin 1986:42(i):3-10.

[3] Neuroscience for kids: Alzheimer's disease.
http://faculty.washington.edu/chudler/alz.html

[4] Alzheimer's 'epidemic' could bankrupt Medicare.
http://www.personalmd.com/news/n0322070411.shtml

[5] Gruenberg EM. The failures of success. Milbank Memorial Fund Quarterly Health and Society 1977;55(1):3-24.

[6] Gruenberg EM, Hagnell O, Ojesjo L, Mitelman M. The rising prevalence of

chronic brain syndrome in the elderly. Paper presented at the Symposium on Society, Stress and Disease: Aging and Old Age, Stockholm, Sweden cited in: Henderson AS. The epidemiology of Alzheimer's disease. British Medical Bulletin 1986:42(i):3.

[7] European Institute of Women's Health. Dementia Care. http://www.eurohealth.ie/remind/intro.htm.

[8] Katzman R, Aronson M, Fuld P, Kawas C, Brown T, Morgenstern H, Frishman W, Gidez L, Elder H, Ooi WL. Development of dementing illnesses in an 80-year-old volunteer cohort. Annals of Neurology,1989;25(4):317-24.

[9] Hoffer A, Walker M. Smart Nutrients: Prevent and Treat Alzheimer's and Senility, Enhance Brain Function and Longevity. Ridgefield, CT: Vital Health Publishing, 2002.

[10] Hoffer A. Niacin Therapy in Psychiatry. Springfield, IL: CC Thomas, 1962.

[11] Morris MC, Evans DA, Bienias PA, Scherr A, Tangney CC, Hebert LE, Bennett DA, Wilson RS, Aggarwal N. Dietary niacin and the risk of incident Alzheimer's disease and of cognitive decline. J Neurology, Psychiatry 2004;75:1093-99.

[12] Foster HD. What Really Causes Alzheimer's Disease. Victoria, BC: Trafford Publishing, 2004.

[13] Hoffer A. Niacin Therapy in Psychiatry. Springfield, IL: CC Thomas, 1962.

[14] Hoffer A. Senility is a form of chronic malnutrition. Report of a National Conference on The Crisis in Health Care for the Aging, sponsored by the Huxley Institute of Biosocial Research, New York, March 6, 1972.

[15] Wysong, P. High HDL cholesterol may protect against dementia. The Medical Post August 10, 2004; 40:9.

[16] Hoffer A. Editorial: "Toxic Vitamins." Journal of Orthomolecular Medicine 2003;18: 123-125.

[17] Hoffer A. Side effects of over-the-counter drugs. Journal of Orthomolecular Medicine 2003;18:168-72.

[18] Bobkova NV. The impact of mineral ascorbates on memory loss. Paper presented at the III World Congress on Vitamin C. Victoria, BC: Committee for World Health, 2001.

[20] Bobkova NV, Nesterova IV, Dana E, Nesterov VI, Aleksandrova IIu, Medvinskaia NI, Samokhia AN. Morpho-functional changes of neurons in temporal cortex in comparison with spatial memory in bulbectomized mice after treatment with minerals and ascorbates. [Russian] Morfologiia, 2003;123(3),27-31.

[21] Engelhart MJ, Geerlings MI, Ruitenberg A, van Swieten JC, Hofman A, Witteman JC. Dietary intake of antioxidants and risk of Alzheimer's disease: Food for thought. Journal of the American Medical Association 2002;287(24):3223-29.

[24] Barberger-Gateau P, Letenneur L, Deschamps V, Pérès K, Jean-François Dartigues JF, Renaud S. Fish, meat, and risk of dementia: Cohort study. British Medical Journal 2002;325:932-33.

[25] MacIsaac R. Mary MacIsaac. Died Age 112. In press, J of Orthomolecular Medicine 2007; 22(2).

[26] Hoffer A, Walker M. Smart Nutrients: Prevent and Treat Alzheimer's and Senility, Enhance Brain Function and Longevity. Ridgefield, CT: Vital Health Publishing, 2002.

STRESS, ANXIETY, AND FATIGUE

Prevalence

Stress costs the United States approximately $300 billion annually because of its adverse impacts on industrial and organizational production. A stressed worker requires about $600 more annually to employ than an unstressed one. This figure of $300 billion does not include any personal, family, or community costs.[1] If, in addition to stress reduction techniques, American and other workers were given extra niacin, this financial loss could be enormously reduced. Patients suffering from stress-related anxiety, depression, and chronic fatigue patients are very common. Many of them have sub-clinical pellagra and would, therefore, respond much better to vitamin B-3 than to the anti-depressants commonly prescribed.

General Adaptation Syndrome

Dr Hans Selye identified stress as a threat to the well-being of any organism.[2,3] This threat can be psychological or physical or both. The body reacts to both in the same way. According to Selye's General Adaptation Syndrome, there are three stress-related phases:

- Alarm phase: This occurs at the first encounter. Stress hormones are poured into the body.
- Adaptation phase: The body has apparently adapted to this stressor and appears to have been successful in so doing, but draws heavily upon its resources to maintain this steady state.
- Exhaustion phase: This can lead ultimately the death of the organism.

In the first phase, the glands are activated and the adrenal cortex releases corticosteroid hormones, while the medulla releases noradrenaline. In the second phase, the adrenal medulla pours both adrenaline and noradrenaline into the blood stream. This release of adrenaline and noradrenaline precipitates a host of other biochemical reactions, designed to help the body deal with stress.

When a cougar chases a rabbit, for example, both animals are under severe stress. If the cougar does not run fast or skillfully enough, it misses its meal. Both animals are programmed to try their utmost. Both animals secrete the catechol amines, blood pressure rises, blood is diverted from the internal organs to the muscles, breathing rate increases, and the sweat glands become more active as both animals concentrate on their main task, survival.

However, adrenaline is very toxic, and if allowed to remain circulating in the body at high levels, it will increase blood pressure and eventually kill the animal. Chronic adrenaline secretion, at low levels, also has numerous deleterious effects. These include mood disorders (depression, mourning, anxiety, fear, and anger) with cardiovascular consequences.[4] Depression also worsens the outlook for coronary heart disease, increasing myocardial infarction, stroke, and carotid atherosclerosis. Anger increases coronary artery disease, premature coronary artery disease, myocardial infarction, and hypertension. These adverse side effects of adrenaline are very dangerous. Contrary activity, which decreases the intensity of such emotions, is therapeutic.

Severe muscular activity and exhaustion depletes the body of adrenaline, and after the 'survival' run, both animals seem to be relatively unconcerned over what has happened. With humans the situation is usually different. If the stress is psychological, the same reactions occur in the body as if it was physical, but, at the end of the episode of anxiety or stress, the body has yet to deal with the excess adrenaline. This it does by rapidly changing adrenaline's structure, using about four different mechanisms, including the formation of adrenochrome.

Role of Vitamin B-3

Niacin is involved in this process because it is invoked in the reactions to stress. This vitamin prevents the release of free fatty acids from the fatty acid storage sites when an animal is exposed to stress. If this process is not inhibited in time, it will lead to increased levels of triglycerides in the blood, higher levels of cholesterol, and eventually serious cardiovascular risk. It is known that rats subjected to stress experience increased levels of blood cholesterol and triglycerides. A Californian study showed that in accountants, the levels of these lipids rose before tax deadlines, showing the extreme sensitivity of lipid level to stress.

Clinical Evidence

Dr E. Cheraskin, a famous orthomolecular physician and dentist, used the *Cornell Medical Index* to show that dental students with higher intakes of niacin in their foods had lower scores, indicating that they were healthier and less stressed.[5] In Sweden, Lars A. Carlson at the King Gustaf V Research Institute showed conclusively that niacin prevented the release of fatty acids, whether the stress was psychological or physical.[6] He found that psychological stress was much less harmful and subjects were calmer if they previously had been given high doses of niacin.

They were also protected physically. When tested after being stressed, patients' adrenaline blood levels were high, but their lipid levels had not increased. If they were not given niacin prior to being exposed to stress, there was a major increase in low density lipoprotein cholesterol.

Niacin elevates HDL, which is advantageous in dealing with stress. One of the best tests of the protective effect of niacin against stress is induced ulcers in rats. Almost all rats placed in restraint develop stress stomach ulcers. Even rats subjected to the same stress but given tranquilizers still develop the same ulcers. However, when they were given niacin, they were totally protected against the side-effects of stress and none developed stomach ulcers.

Stress and Surgery

Although modern anesthetics and new technologies have reduced the pain and suffering of surgery, it is still an extremely stressful experience. The early use of niacin has a very beneficial effect on arteries, brain, and heart, and, if widely used, could reduce the number of patients requiring surgery. Beyond this, it has been shown that two anti-oxidants, vitamin E and ascorbic acid, in high doses, can reduce the incidence of organ failure during surgery and shorten the length of stay required by critically ill surgical patients in the Intensive Care Units.[7] Clinical trials of the use of niacin before and after surgery seem warranted.

Malnutrition and Stress

Oxidative stress plays a key role in many diseases and in the aging process itself. Its impact, however, is magnified by malnutrition, the deficiency of a variety of nutrients, including those that protect the body against oxidative stress. The adverse impacts of combined stress and malnutrition peaked in the concentration camps in Europe and the prisoner of war camps in the Far East during the Second World War. To illustrate, Dr Hans Selye used death rates to quantify stress in animal experiments. If it killed as many as 10% of those animals involved, then stress was considered to have been very severe. Yet more than 90% of the prisoners in Europe's concentration camps were killed and up to 50% of soldiers captured and held prisoner in Japanese POW camps also died.

The effects of this stress-malnutrition combination did not end upon release. Its subsequent impacts were obvious on the aging process.[8,9] More than 2,000 untrained Canadian soldiers were sent to Hong Kong to defend it from invasion from the east, but the Japanese attacked from the west, and soon these Canadian soldiers were captured and placed in prison camps. Forty-four months later, one quarter of them had died, and the rest were left permanently impaired. On their way home in hospital ships, they were fed the strongest vitamin preparation then available, rice bran extracts, and they rapidly began to regain their health. Those who had survived had lost up to one third of their body weight and began to replace some of this loss.

Although they appeared to become well again, they did not. A survey conducted by the federal government established that they were much sicker than Canadian soldiers who had fought in Europe, and, as a result, they were given special pensions. After the war, they suffered to an exaggerated degree from all the diseases of aging, including arthritis, blindness, heart disease, neurological deterioration, and depression. Dr Hoffer estimated that one year in a Japanese POW camp aged these soldiers about 5 years, as compared to a normal year living at home. A soldier imprisoned in such a camp at chronological age 35 would come out 4 years later with a biological age of 55.

Former prisoners of war began to suffer predictably after their release. Initial after-effects generally lasted from 1947 to 1955, with chronic fatigue being the main symptom. A second phase followed, consisting mainly of deterioration of the cardiovascular and the central nervous system.

One of these former Hong Kong veterans was the administrator of a retirement home for many elderly men and women. Dr Hoffer was studying the effect of niacin on the aging process, and this veteran wanted to try it himself, so that he could discuss the associated flush more intelligently with the retirement home residents. Later, he described his 44-month experience in the Far East prison camp to Dr Hoffer and explained how sick he had been after coming back to Canada.

He had been depressed, experienced severe arthritis, was fearful, was heat and cold intolerant, and had spent some time on a psychiatric ward for veterans. He had been diagnosed as having a personality disorder. Much to his surprise, after 2 weeks on niacin, he became normal. All his symptoms disappeared. He became Lieutenant Governor for the Province of Saskatchewan and remained well until he died years later.

Through his intercession, 20 more Hong Kong veterans, as well as American former prisoners of war, came to see Dr Hoffer for treatment. Given niacin, they all recovered. The high dose niacin reversed the health deterioration caused by the extraordinarily severe stress of these camps.

Even without brutality and mental torture, life-threatening malnutrition is very stressful. Its effects from one generation to another tend to be cumulative. The effect of this intergenerational deprivation has been demonstrated in animals. Feeding rats an inadequate diet, generation after generation, will lead to increasing psychological and physical ill health.

Even moderate transgenerational under-nutrition has a cumulative effect in impairing neurocranial and facial growth in rats.[10] When rats that had been under-nourished for many generations were placed upon an adequate diet, it took several generations before their offspring returned to normal. This may be a model of what is happening to human health today.

In industrialized nations, the population is not calorie deficient, but it is deprived of adequate micro-nutrients. The quality of human food has been deteriorating for many years with serious health implications. As seen in animal studies and in prisoners of war, it is not easy to recover from long-term nutritional deficiencies.

On a global scale, these adverse health implications may take as much as a century to correct. In the developing world, many people are suffering from massive calorie deficiencies, in addition to a general micro-nutrient inadequacy. Indeed, the world is threatened by ongoing pandemics of HIV/AIDS, hepatitis B and C, tuberculosis, and, potentially, avian influenza that are being driven by the mineral impoverishment of global soils and the poorer quality food they are producing. Professor Foster has described, for example, the role played by selenium deficiency in accelerating the HIV/AIDS pandemic.[11,12]

Anti-aging

Niacin is a remarkable anti-aging nutrient, much simpler and safer than drugs prescribed to treat aging conditioned. A study by L.H. Curtis and colleagues concluded that out of a sample of 162,370 elderly subjects, 21% were given prescriptions for one or more drugs that were considered inappropriate.[13] More than 15% of them had prescriptions for two of such drugs, and 4% were getting three or more. Curtis was concerned because of the potential for severe side effects. Dr Hoffer recently met with one elderly patient who was taking 28 different drugs, all on prescription. When orthomolecular medicine is practiced and nutrients, such as niacin, are used, the potential for dangerous side effects is greatly reduced. It will no longer be true that "Our elderly are adrift in a sea of drugs."[14]

Anxiety

In 2005, Dr Jonathan E. Prousky described three patients suffering from anxiety disorder, who greatly improved when prescribed 2,000 to 2,500 mg of niacinamide on a daily basis.[15] Each of these patients found considerable relief from anxiety with regular use of this vitamin. Prousky put forward several possible reasons for this response: the correction of subclinical pellagra; an underlying vitamin B-3 dependency disorder; and the ability of niacinamide to raise serotonin levels and modify the metabolism of blood lactate (lactic acid). Subsequently, Prousky expanded his research results in his book, *Anxiety: Orthomolecular Diagnosis and Treatment*.[16]

References

[1] Schwartz J. Always at work and anxious employees' health is suffering. The New York Times, Sunday, September 5, 2004.

[2] Selye HHB. The Stress of Life. New York, NY: McGrawHill, 1956.

[3] Selye HHB. Stress without Distress. Philadelphia, PA: JB Lippincott Co., 1974.

[4] Anderson RA. Psychoneuroimmunoendocrinology review and commentary. Townsend Letter for Doctors and Patients 2004 August/September;253:254.

[5] Cheraskin E. How quickly does diet make for change? A study of weight in dental students. J. Ala Dent Assoc 1988;72(3):28-31.

[6] Carlson LA. Nicotinic acid: The broad-spectrum lipid drug. A 50th anniversary review. J Intern Med 2005;258(2):94-114.

[7] Natheens AB, Neff MJ, Jurkovich MD, et al. Randomized prospective trial of antioxidant supplementation in critically ill surgical patients. Annals of Surgery 2002; 236:814-22.

[8] Hoffer A. Hong Kong veterans study. J Orthomolecular Psychiatry 1974;3:34-36.

[9] Hoffer A. Senility and chronic malnutrition. J Orthomolecular Psychiatry 1974;3:2-19.

[10] Cesani MF, Orden B, Zucchi M, Mune MC, Oyhenart EE, and Pucciarelli HM. Effect of undernutrition on the cranial growth of the rat. Cell Tissue Organs 2003;174:129-35.

[11] Foster HD. Why HIV-1 has diffused so much more rapidly in sub-Saharan Africa than in North America. Medicine Hypotheses 2003;60(4):611-14.

[12] Foster HD. Halting the AIDS pandemic. In: Janelle DG, Warf B, Hansen K (eds). WorldMinds: Geographical Perspectives on 100 Problems. Dordrecht: Kluwer Academic Publishers, 2004:69-73.

[13] Curtis LH, Ostbye T, Sendersky V, Hutchison S, Dans PE, Wright A, Woosley RL, Schulman KA. Inappropriate prescribing for elderly Americans in a large outpatient population. Archives Internal Medicine 2004;164:1621-25.

[14] Picard A. Our elderly are adrift in a sea of drugs. Toronto, ON: The Globe and Mail, June 3, 2004.

[15] Prousky JE. Supplemental niacinamide mitigates anxiety symptoms: Three case reports. J Orthomolecular Medicine 2005;20(3):167-78.

[16] Prousky JE. Anxiety: Orthomolecular Diagnosis and Treatment. Toronto, ON: CCNM Press Inc., 2006.

CANCER

Prevalence

In the United States, malignant neoplasms are the dominant cause of death among those aged 45 to 64 years, being replaced by heart disease and dropping to the second most common cause of mortality in the more elderly.[1] In total, roughly one million Americans are now developing cancer each year, and about 500,000 are dying from it.[2] According to Health Canada and the Canadian Cancer Society, about 40% of Canadian men and 35% of women will develop cancer during their lifetimes.[3] Indeed, 25% of all Canadian men and 20% of women will die from it.

Role of Vitamin B-3

There can be no doubt that nutrition plays an important role in determining who develops cancer.[4-7] Many nutrients, including calcium and selenium, appear to protect against specific malignant neoplasms.[8-9] This also appears to be true of vitamin B-3, which has anti-cancer properties. In 1987, for example, Dr M. Jacobson and Dr E. Jacobson presented a paper at The Eighth International Symposium on ADP-Ribosylation, held in Fort Worth, Texas, that discussed "Niacin, nutrition, ADP-ribosylation and cancer."[10]

Niacin, niacinamide, and nicotinamide adenine dinucleotide (NAD) are inter-convertible via a pyridine nucleotide cycle. NAD, the coenzyme, is hydrolyzed or split into niacinamide and adenosine dinucleotide phosphate (ADP-ribose). Niacinamide is converted into niacin, which in turn is once more built into NAD. The enzyme that splits ADP is known as poly (ADP-ribose) polymerase, poly (ADP) synthetase, or poly (ADP-ribose) transferase.

Poly (ADP-ribose) polymerase is activated when strands of deoxyribonucleic acid (DNA) are broken. The enzyme transfers NAD to the ADP-ribose polymer, binding it onto a number of proteins. The poly (ADP-ribose) activated by DNA breaks helps repair such breaks by unwinding the nucleosomal structure of damaged chromatids. It also may increase the activity of DNA ligase. This enzyme cuts damaged ends off strands of DNA and increases the cells capacity to repair itself. Damage caused by any carcinogenic factor, such as radiation or chemicals is, as a result, neutralized or counteracted.

Jacobson and Jacobson hypothesized that this is why niacin can protect against cancer. They illustrated this by treating two groups of human cells with carcinogens. The group given adequate niacin developed tumors at a rate of only 10% of that seen in what was deficient in niacin. Dr M. Jacobson is quoted as saying, "We know that diet is a major risk factor, that diet has both beneficial and detrimental components. What we cannot assess at this point is the optimal amount of niacin in the diet. ...The fact that we don't have pellagra does not mean we are getting enough niacin to confer resistance to cancer."[11] Further evidence of niacin's anti-cancer role has been provided by K. Titus and by D. Hostetler. [12,13]

Clinical Evidence

Dr Max Gerson treated a series of cancer patients with special diets and with nutrients, including niacin (50 mg, 8 to 10 times per day), dicalcium phosphate, vitamins A and D, and liver injections.[14] He found that all of these patients benefited. That is, they became healthier and in many cases their tumors regressed. In a subsequent report, Gerson elaborated on his diet.[15] He emphasized high potassium and low sodium and supplements of ascorbic acid, brewer's yeast, Lugol's iodine, and niacin. In the late 1940s, there was no ready supply of vitamins, and the use of these nutrients in combination was very original and enterprising. Dr Gerson appears to have been the first physician to emphasize the use of multivitamins and some multiminerals in the treatment of cancer.

Vitamin B-3 may increase the therapeutic efficacy of more traditional anti-cancer treatment. E. Kjellen and coworkers, for example, gave mice niacinamide, at a rate of 0.2 g per kg of body weight, 30 minutes before they were given radiation.[16] One week earlier they had been injected with mammary adenocarcinoma cells. This dose of vitamin B-3 is equivalent to 12 g per day of niacinamide for an average human adult. The vitamin B-3 had no direct effect on tumor volume in these animals; however, it decreased 86% after irradiation in niacinamide-treated mice, and remained 79% lower at 4 weeks. Mitotic activity also remained low in niacinamide-treated animals after irradiation, but returned to pre-irradiation levels in non-treated mice. Kjellen suggested, therefore, that niacinamide might have a role in the treatment of malignant tumors.

Other authors also have suggested that niacinamide increases the toxicity of irradiation against tumors in mice. M.R. Horsman and colleagues[17-19] and D.J. Chaplin and coworkers[20] found that nicotinamide was the best drug for increasing sensitivity to radioactivity as compared to a series of analogues. This vitamin probably worked because it enhanced blood flow to the tumor.[21]

Nicotinamide also appears to enhance the effects of chemotherapy.[22] However, it is known that radiotherapy decreases the amount of nicotinamide adenine dinucleotide (NAD) in the liver by impairing the conversion of tryptophan to NAD.[23] Since both niacin and niacinamide are readily incorporated into NAD, it would seem prudent for every patient receiving radiation to take supplemental vitamin B-3. This suggestion also applies to people exposed to irradiation from any other source.

Niacin may play a role in reducing the number of birth defects. H. Gotoh and colleagues, for example, reported that nicotinamide significantly decreased urethane-induced malformations when given intraperitoneally to pregnant mice.[24] Beyond this, M.E. Scheulin and colleagues found that niacin also reduced the negative impacts of adriamycin, a widely used agent in chemotherapy, on the heart.[25] As a result, they suggested that niacin may offer some cardioprotection during long-term adriamycin chemotherapy.

Further evidence that vitamin B-3 deficiency is involved in cancer is provided in a report by K. Nakagawa that in animals there is a direct relationship between the activity of nicotinamide methyl transferase and the presence of cancer.[26] The amount of N-methyl nicotinamide present was used as a measure of the activity of the enzyme. In other words, in animals with cancer, there appears to be an increased destruction of nicotinamide, making less of it available for the pyridine nucleotide cycle. This finding applied to most tumors, except Lewis lung carcinoma and melanoma B-16.

A news release from the University of Guelph, dated March 25, 2003, also supports the belief that niacin prevents treatment-related cancers. Professor James Kirkland reported 47% more cancer treatment-related malignancies in niacin-deficient rats.[27] Chemotherapy damages DNA, not only of the cancer cells, but in developing blood cells in the bone marrow, causing new treatment-related cancers, such as leukemia and cancer of the bone marrow. As a consequence, those undergoing chemotherapy are 10 to 100 times more likely to develop such cancers as the general public, and 3 to 10 times more likely than patients undergoing only radiation. Niacin deficient animals have depleted NAD stores, which in turn are involved in the repair of damaged DNA. It was found that rats given niacin before treatment lived longer. The news release concluded that the "pharmacological supplementation of niacin may represent a rapid and safe way to help protect the bone marrow cells of cancer patients."

Further evidence that niacin may be beneficial as a cancer preventative was provided by the National Coronary Study.[28] During the period 1966 to 1975, 8341 men, aged 30 to 64 years, who had suffered a heart attack at least 3 months earlier, were entered into a study comparing the benefits of five substances normally used to lower cholesterol levels, against a placebo. Nine years later only niacin had decreased the death rate significantly from all causes. Those taking this vitamin showed an 11% decrease in mortality and a 2-year increase in longevity. Interestingly, their cancer mortality rates also had fallen.

In a more recent literature review, it was shown that in spite of fortification of flour with niacinamide, many people are deficient in vitamin B-3, even though they may not show obvious signs of pellagra. In Sweden, 15% of females were found to be deficient in vitamin B-3, while in the United States, 22% of the geriatric population were eating inadequate amounts. In such niacin deficient individuals, genes are more susceptible to DNA damage. In one study reviewed by Spronk and Kirkland, 40% of cancer patients receiving chemotherapy were shown to be niacin deficient.[29] It was concluded that "the basic research reviewed in this article illustrates the potential of niacin status to impact on genomic stability and cancer incidence in human populations." Clearly, it is essential to maintain high enough levels of the enzyme poly (ADP-ribose) polymerase (PARP) to repair damaged DNA. It is not for nothing that this enzyme is called the guardian of the genome. Niacin deficiency decreases PARP activity and so limits DNA damage repair, increasing the chance of developing cancer.

An association between niacin deficiency and cancer has been shown in populations eating low-protein corn diets in Italy and South Africa and in some provinces of China. Tissues vary in their sensitivity to low niacin. Bone marrow is most sensitive. Niacin deficiency, therefore, increases the rate of appearance and number of chemically induced cancers, especially forms of leukemia originating in the bone marrow.

Skin is also very sensitive to niacin deficiency. In rats, a lack of this vitamin increases the production of UV induced skin cancers. Niacin supplements can protect against this type of cancer. Niacin deficiency apparently causes an increase in gross chromosomal instability.

This increase in cancer in the skin of niacin-deficient individuals raises the issue of the link, if any, between exposure to the sun and the development of melanoma. The great majority of dermatologists have accepted that exposure to the sun is the major cause of melanoma. There are exceptions to this generalization. Dr Bernard Ackerman, after reviewing the literature and drawing on his own experience in dermatology, concluded that the connection is both inconclusive and inconsistent.[30] To illustrate, melanoma usually develops in skin that has not been exposed. Ackerman also questions the use of sun screens, and points out that sunburns do not necessarily lead to melanoma. He does advise avoiding excessive exposure to sun, however, to decrease aging of the skin.

Unfortunately, the desire to avoid the sun to prevent the development of skin cancer is leading many people to become vitamin D-3 deficient.

Rickets, a vitamin D-3 deficiency disease is, for example, reappearing in Canada and seems to be averaging about 40 cases a year. Beyond the prevention of rickets, vitamin D-3 is known to have valuable anticancer properties in its own right.

Exposure to the sun should occur in moderation. To avoid excess, it is best to avoid the sun between 10:00 a.m. and 3:00 p.m., to use clothing, to allow only partial exposure, and to be sure to have a high enough intake of vitamin C, vitamin E, selenium, and niacin or niacinamide. Taking extra vitamin D-3 is essential to avoid rickets.[31, 32]

References

[1] Health! Canada Magazine. Cancer: What's your risk?
http://www.hc-sc.gc.ca/english/feature/magazine/2001°04/cancer.htm

[2] Presbyterian Hunger Program. Pesticides. Food and Faith.
http://www.pcusa.org/pcusa/wmd/hunger/food/pesticides.htm

[3] Health! Canada Magazine. Cancer: What's your risk?
http://www.hc-sc.gc.ca/english/feature/magazine/2001°04/cancer.htm

[4] Passwater RA. Cancer and Its Nutritional Therapies. New Canaan, CT: Keats Publishing, Inc., 1978.

[5] Quillin P, Williams RM (eds.) Adjuvant Nutrition in Cancer Treatment. Arlington Heights, IL: Cancer Treatment Research Foundation, 1993:55-79.

[6] Moss RW. Cancer Therapy: The Independent Consumers Guide to Non-Toxic Treatment and Prevention. New York, NY: Equinox Press, 1992.

[7] Simone CVB. Cancer and Nutrition. Garden City Park, NY: Avery Publishing Group, Inc., 1992.

[8] Foster HD. Calcium and cancer: A geographical perspective. Journal of Orthomolecular Medicine 1998;13(3):173-75.

[9] Foster HD. Selenium and cancer: A geographical perspective. Journal of Orthomolecular Medicine 1998;13(1):8-10.

[10] Jacobson M, Jacobson E. Niacin, nutrition, ADP-ribosylation and cancer. The 8th International Symposium on ADP-Ribosylation. Fort Worth, TX: Texas College of Osteopathic Medicine, 1987.

[11] Jacobson M, Jacobson E. Niacin, nutrition, ADP-ribosylation and cancer. The 8th International Symposium on ADP-Ribosylation. Fort Worth, TX: Texas College of Osteopathic Medicine, 1987.

[12] Titus K. Scientists link niacin and cancer prevention. The D.O. 1987; 3-97.

[13] Hostetler D. Jacobsons put broad strokes in the niacin/cancer picture. The D.O. 1987; 3-104.

[14] Gerson M. Dietary considerations in malignant neoplastic disease. A preliminary report. The Review of Gastroenterology 1945;12:419-25.

[15] Gerson M. Effects of a combined dietary regime on patients with malignant tumors. Experimental Medicine and Surgery 1949;7:299-317.

[16] Kjellen E, Pero RW, Cameron R, Ranstam J. Radiosensitizing effects of nicotinamide on a C3H mouse mammary adenocarcinoma. Acta Radiologica Oncology 1986;25:281-284.

[17] Horsman MR, Chaplin DJ, Brown JM. Tumor radiosensitization by nicotinamide: A result of improved perfusion and oxygenation. Radiation Research 1989;118:139-50.

[19] Horsman PE, Kristjansen MR, Mizuno M, Christensen KL, Chaplin DJ, Quistorff B, Overgaard J. Biochemical and physiological changes induced by nicotinamide in   a C3H mouse mammary carcinoma and CDF1 mice. Int J Radiation Oncology, Biology, Physics 1992;22:451-54.

[20] Chaplin DJ, Horsman MP, and Aoki DS. Nicotinamide, fluosol DA and carbogen: A strategy to reoxygenate acutely and chronically hypoxic cells in vivo. British Journal of Cancer 1990;63:109-113.

[21] Horsman MR, Chaplin DJ, Brown JM. Tumor radiosensitization by nicotinamide: A result of improved perfusion and oxygenation. Radiation Research 1989;118:139-50.

[22] Chen G, Pan QC. Potentiation of the antitumor activity of cisplatin in mice

by 3-aminobenzamide and nicotinamide. Cancer Chemotherapy and Pharmacology 1988;22: 303-307.

23 Streffer C. The biosynthesis of NAD in the liver of irradiated mice. J of Vitaminology 1968;14:130-34.

24 Gotoh H, Nomura T, Nakajima C, Hasegawa C, Sakamoto Y. Inhibiting effects of nicotinamide on urethane-induced malformations and tumors in mice. Mutation Research 1988;199:55-63.

25 Scheulin ME, Schmitt-Graff A, Schmidt CG. Reduction of adriamycin cardiotoxicity by niacin and isocitrate. Proc 74th Ann Meeting, Amer. Assoc. Cancer Research 1983;24:251.

26 Nakagawa K, Miyazaka M, Okui K, Kato N, Moriyama Y, and Fujimura S. N-methylnicotinamide level in the blood after nicotinamide loading as further evidence for malignant tumor burden. Jap. J Cancer Research 1991; 82:1277-83.

27 Kirkland J. Department of Human Biology and Nutrition Science. \jkirklan@uoguelph.ca

28 Canner PL, Berge KG, Wenger NK, Stamler J, Friedman L, Prineas RJ, Freidewald W. Fifteen year mortality coronary drug project: Patients long term benefit with niacin. American College of Cardiology 1986; 8:1245-55.

29 Spronk JC, Kirkland JB. Niacin status, poly (ADP-ribose) metabolism and genomic instability. In. Zempleni J, Daniel (eds) Molecular Nutrition. Wallingford, UK: CAB International 2003.

30 Ackerman AB. Gina kolata. New York Times, July 20, 2004.

31 Burke KE. Oral and topical L-selenomethionine protection from ultraviolet-induced sunburn, tanning and skin cancer. Journal Orthomolecular Medicine, 1992;7:83-94.

32 Burke KE, Combs GF Jr, Gross EG, et al. The effects of topical and oral L-selenomethionine on pigmentation and skin cancer induced by ultraviolet irradiation. Nutrition and Cancer, 1992;17:123-33.

Risks and Benefits

As with any form of therapy, vitamin B-3 needs to be evaluated on the basis of its risks and benefits. In a recent issue of the *Journal of Orthomolecular Medicine*, Dr Hoffer has reviewed the literature on the negative and positive side effects of vitamin B-3.[1,2] Despite early concerns about the safety of niacin therapy in the medical literature, subsequent studies have shown it to be remarkably safe, especially when compared to the risks involved with drug treatments for the same conditions. When first ingested in large doses, niacin has a discomfiting vasodilation or flushing effect, which typically subsides after steady use or can be avoided with the use of niacinamide. This side effect is, in fact, a side benefit in many cases, for example, in patients suffering from arthritis and high cholesterol levels.

Liver Toxicity

Between 1940 and 1950, when the toxicity of niacin and niacinamide was first studied, the LD_{50} for rats was determined – the amount, if given as one dose, that would kill 50% of the test animals. It was very high, about 4.5 g per kg. However, at autopsy, the animals showed elevated fatty acid in the liver.

In 1950, a deficiency of methyl groups was known to cause fatty livers. Niacin and niacinamide are methyl acceptors. It made sense, therefore, to consider the possibility that too much vitamin B-3 caused fatty acid livers by producing a methyl deficiency syndrome. Some experiments suggested this was so, but when these experiments were repeated by Professor R. Altschul of the University of Saskatchewan, the results did not confirm these findings.[3] In his animal studies, he found that vitamin B-3 had no effect on the fatty acid levels in the liver.

Vitamin B-3 has also been associated with increased liver function tests in some patients.[4] This may be so, but elevated liver function tests do not always means underlying liver pathology. Many harmless substances have the same effect. Mayo Clinic researchers examined the livers of a series of their patients who were receiving niacin for high blood cholesterol. Even using the electro microscope, they could find no evidence of pathology. This negative finding was first reported by Dr W. Parsons Jr., who pointed out that increased liver function tests, unless they are very substantial (more than three-fold normal), do not indicate liver pathology.

There are many compounds that elevate liver enzymes, including all the statin drugs. In most patients with elevated liver function, test values become normal in a few days, even if the niacin is not discontinued. In one study, J. Gonzalez-Heydrich and colleagues gave 12 children a combination of olanzapine and divalproic acid.[5] All had an elevated enzyme peak, which in five of them remained present for many months. Two children had to be removed from the study because of severe pathology, pancreatitis in one case, and steatohepatitis in the other.

It is possible that the liver function tests may be increased by high doses of niacin due to methyl depletion. According to Professor David Capuzzi, one of the world's authorities on niacin and cholesterol, this potential problem can be prevented by giving patients 1 or 2 grams of lecithin in the morning and again at night.[6] Betaine may also be effective in this protective role.

Dr Hoffer advises all doctors who refer patients to him that they should stop niacin therapy for at least 5 days before liver function tests are conducted.

With real liver pathology, these tests will not be normal in 5 days, but when results are elevated by niacin, they return to normal within 5 days.

More than 40 years ago, there were a few reports of liver damage and one or two deaths reported from high niacin intake. These were traced to poorly-made, slow-release preparations, but never were found associated with standard preparations.

Dr Hoffer has used niacin for lowering cholesterol and both niacin and niacinamide for treating thousands of schizophrenic patients since 1953. A few cases of jaundice occurred in early patients, which might have been due to impure niacin preparations. Some bottles of niacin had a pyridine smell. But jaundice was rare and has not occurred for decades. One patient recovering from schizophrenia on niacin became jaundiced, but when the niacin was stopped, the jaundice cleared. However, his schizophrenia returned. When the niacin was restarted, his schizophrenia cleared again and jaundice did not recur. There have been no similar cases in the past 20 years.

Side Effects

There are some minor side effects of high dose vitamin B-3 that may be a nuisance, but are not toxic reactions. Apart from a very few people who are allergic to this supplement, either due to its active component or to some of the commonly used fillers, most adverse reactions are dose related.

Most negative side effects occur very infrequently at smaller dose levels, only becoming more common with higher doses. These side effects result from niacin intake, not niacinamide. For example, enriching the food supply so it provides 100 mg of niacinamide daily is not noticed by the average consumer. However, taking large doses of niacin does have a discomfiting but not dangerous effect because of vasodilation or 'flush' when first taken. The flush associated with niacin is 'dry', unlike the menopausal flush or the flush created by male hormone blockers used in treating prostate cancer. The higher the initial dose, the greater the flush. However, there is a threshold dose, which, if maintained, does not cause any more flushing unless the niacin is not taken regularly. The dose is usually 1 g taken three times (after three meals), but, in some cases, it may have to be as high as 3 g taken three times daily.

Niacin usually causes a flush a few minutes after it is taken. Some people will flush given a 25-mg dose, more with 50, and most with 100 mg. If niacin is taken regularly, the flush is repeated, but to a much lesser degree. In most cases, after a week or so, it is greatly reduced and has become a minor nuisance at worst. The intensity of the flush can be minimized by taking the pills regularly after meals, three times daily. If niacin is not taken for a few days, the flush will recur.

The flush begins in the forehead and works its way down the body, rarely affecting the toes. Flushing occurs as the capillaries are dilated and the blood flow through the organs is increased. There is also an internal increase in blood flow, as well as in the skin. This may last up to several hours. For many people, the vasodilatation is very beneficial because it increases the flow of blood to almost all the tissues.

Patients taking niacin for the first time must be warned that this will happen. If not, they may be very surprised and even shocked. An internist treating patients with niacin one day forgot to advise his patient. When his patient took his first dose and flushed, he was so fearful he promptly called the poison control center of the nearest hospital. The person who answered the phone obviously knew nothing about niacin and told him he had taken a lethal dose and sent an ambulance. By the time the ambulance arrived at the hospital, the flush was over.

Some people do not stop flushing. They should discontinue taking the niacin because the flushing is very irritating and may cause skin lesions. Non-flush preparations, such as niacinamide and inositol niacinate, are available in these cases. Niacinamide normally does not cause any flushing, except in about 1% of the population. These people experience a very unpleasant flush, and should not use it. It seems likely that they are converting the niacinamide too rapidly into niacin.

Other uncommon side effects of niacin are increased gastric acidity, probably caused by niacin stimulation of secretion of gastric juice, and increased brown pigmentation of certain areas of the skin, usually the flexor surfaces. This is not acanthosis nigricans. The niacin reaction is a skin change that resembles acanthosis nigricans, but only in color, not in pathology. This rare browning effect of niacin is transient, usually lasting only a few months, and when it clears, the skin is perfectly normal. Like an old tan, it washes off if the skin is rubbed when moist. The condition never recurs, even with continued niacin use. The pigmentation is never a problem for patients if they are well-informed.

The cause of this browning effect may be due to the deposition of melanin-containing indoles from tyrosine and adrenaline. Not surprisingly, it occurs most commonly in schizophrenic patients and can be seen as a marker in the healing process. Many years ago, Dr Hoffer treated a mute female schizophrenic patient. After a few months in hospital, she improved and was discharged. After discharge, Dr Hoffer saw her and her husband monthly. At one of these meetings about 3 months later, Dr Hoffer felt that she was ready to talk and asked her how she felt. In response, she began to talk. Suddenly, she stretched out both of her hands, displaying her fingers. The distal half of each nail was a dirty yellow-brown color and the proximal half was a clear and healthy nail. Her toenails were similar. Apparently, a few months after depositing pigment, she was well enough to start talking once more. This patient's case history clearly demonstrates the presence of a schizophrenic toxin, which is a melanin-like-substance, derived from adrenochrome or adrenolutin.

Side Benefits

Most of the side effects of high dose niacin are positive. Vasodilatation is sometimes very helpful. Many patients, particularly arthritics, have reported that they feel much better when their joints are warmed up by the niacin flush. Some will stop taking niacin for a few days in order to reactivate it.

There are many physical and psychiatric diseases that benefit from niacin. When these are being treated, there will, of course, be other positive side effects. If a patient, for example, takes niacin to normalize blood lipids and, as a result of the vitamin activity, feels very much better, displaying more energy or faster healing, these are positive side effects. If a patient takes niacin to deal with arthritis, but at the same time it causes a decline in cholesterol levels, this is a major positive side effect – or side benefit.

Conclusion

V itamins are universally considered safe. Niacin has not been proven to cause liver damage. Liver disease is relatively common, and by coincidence, a person with developing liver problems may also have been taking niacin. The benefits of niacin are so great and the relatively minor side effects so slight that there can be no question of its safety. It is probably more dangerous not to take niacin.

References

[1] Hoffer A. Niacin Therapy in Psychiatry. Springfield IL: CC Thomas, 1962.

[2] Hoffer A. Negative and positive side effects of vitamin B-3. Journal of Orthomolecular Medicine 2003;18:146-60.

[3] Altschul R. Personal communication.

[4] Parsons WB Jr. Cholesterol Control Without Diet. The Niacin Solution. Revised, Expanded, 2nd ed. Scottsdale, AZ: Lilac Press, 2003.

[5] Gonzalez-Heydrich J. Wilens RD, Leichtner A, Messacappa E. Retrospective study of hepatic enzyme elevations in children treated with olanzapine, divalproic acid and their combination. J American Academy Child Adolescent Psychiatry 2003;42:1227-33.

[6] Cappuzi D. 2002 Personal communication.

Acknowledgments

To Professor D. G. McKerracher, Director Psychiatric Services Branch, Department of Public Health, Province of Saskatchewan, and Premier Tommy Douglas for having created the research division in 1950.

To Dr Humphry Osmond and Dr John Smythies for introducing the trans-methylation idea into psychiatry, which led to our adrenochrome hypothesis, which, in turn, led to the use of high doses of vitamin B-3 and ascorbic acid for treating schizophrenia.

To M. J. Callbeck, Research Nurse, for ensuring that the clinical records and protocols were conducted properly.

To Dr Arthur Sackler for publishing our first report on the treatment of schizophrenia with vitamin B-3, 1957,

To all the members of the Saskatchewan Committee on Schizophrenia Research who supervised and supported this research from 1950 to 1965.

To Luella who joined the Hoffer household after 17 years in a chronic mental hospital and allowed him to learn what it means to be schizophrenic.

To all the doctors who rejected the false belief that niacin is dangerous.

To the thousands of patients who have willingly helped us understand what it is like to be sick and how it can be treated by non-toxic means.

To Dr Linus Pauling for his tremendous support and for establishing the term orthomolecular, the most accurate description of the method for using natural products that are normally present in the body. After 40 years of rejection, scientific acceptance is advancing rapidly.

To all the pioneers, listed in the Orthomolecular Hall of Fame.

To Fran Fuller and J. Mawdsley for typing and editorial help.

To Sarah Foster for proofreading this book.

To Andrew W. Saul who has been so successful in educating the public with his extraordinarily accurate and widely read web site www.doctoryourself.com

To Steven Carter for his tremendous support of the principles and practices of orthomolecular medicine and the vast importance of vitamin B-3.

To Bob Hilderley and his staff at CCNM Press for their very helpful editing and publishing of this book.